320
Single Best Answer Questions for Final Year Medical Students
Second Edition

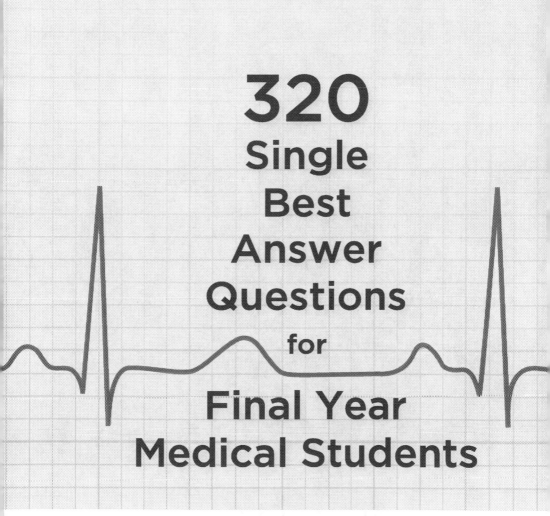

320
Single
Best
Answer
Questions
for
Final Year
Medical Students

Second Edition

Adam Ioannou
Royal Free Hospital, UK

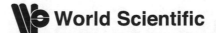

World Scientific

Published by

World Scientific Publishing Co. Pte. Ltd.

5 Toh Tuck Link, Singapore 596224

USA office: 27 Warren Street, Suite 401-402, Hackensack, NJ 07601

UK office: 57 Shelton Street, Covent Garden, London WC2H 9HE

Library of Congress Cataloging-in-Publication Data

Names: Ioannou, Adam, author.

Title: 320 single best answer questions for final year medical students / Adam Ioannou.

Description: Second edition. | New Jersey : World Scientific, [2020]

Identifiers: LCCN 2019032258| ISBN 9789811210082 (hardcover) |
    ISBN 9789811210778 (paperback)

Subjects: | MESH: Medicine | Students, Medical | Examination Question

Classification: LCC R834.5 | NLM WB 18.2 | DDC 610.76--dc23

LC record available at https://lccn.loc.gov/2019032258

British Library Cataloguing-in-Publication Data

A catalogue record for this book is available from the British Library.

For any available supplementary material, please visit
https://www.worldscientific.com/worldscibooks/10.1142/11544#t=suppl

Typeset by Stallion Press

Email: enquiries@stallionpress.com

Printed in Singapore

About the Author

Adam Ioannou studied undergraduate medicine at University College London, and during his third year was awarded a Bachelor of Science in Medical Sciences with Physiology with First Class Honours. He qualified in 2015 with a Bachelor of Medicine and Bachelor of Surgery; and was awarded distinctions in both Clinical Science and Clinical Practice for placing in the top 10% of medical students in the end of year examinations. Since qualifying he has published multiple original research papers, review papers and case reports. He completed his Membership of the Royal College of Physicians exams in 2018, and is currently working as a cardiology registrar in London.

Preface

Single best answer style questions are the most popular means of written assessment in both undergraduate and postgraduate medical examinations. Each clinical vignette is followed by a list of five possible answers, of which there is one that is the most clinically appropriate. The questions are designed to test the candidates' medical knowledge and their ability to apply this to clinical scenarios, rather than just their capability to recall facts.

The 320 questions are divided into 11 commonly tested areas of medicine, surgery and sub-specialities. The questions are written in the same format as those in medical school exams and are designed to provide a comprehensive coverage of the medical school curriculum.

This improved edition contains updated and new questions that are in line with the most recent developments in clinical guidelines as well as being written in accordance with the recent changes to medical school examinations. It also contains a proportion of harder stems that are designed to challenge the reader and help the student reach their maximum potential. The more challenging questions push the reader to think through various aspects of the topic being tested; requiring a multi-step thought process to reach the correct answer. This type of questioning is becoming increasingly popular in medical school examinations.

The answers provide detailed explanations as to how the correct answer is reached, followed by a clear discussion of how the incorrect answers are ruled out and supplementary information about other important aspects of each question.

Progression through each section will allow the reader to grow and develop their single best answer technique, as well as acquire useful knowledge and understanding that is needed during clinical practice; a combination of which will leave the reader well prepared for medical exams.

Good luck with your examination preparation.

Contents

Cardiology Questions

1. A 65-year-old man with a previous history of tuberculosis presents to clinic feeling short of breath and complaining of ankle swelling. He is currently stable and his blood pressure is 130/90 mmHg. On examination it is noticed that his jugular venous pressure (JVP) rises on inspiration. What is the underlying diagnosis?

A. Tricuspid regurgitation
B. Cardiac tamponade
C. Constrictive pericarditis
D. Pulmonary hypertension
E. Dilated cardiomyopathy

2. A 78-year-old woman who has been diagnosed with multiple myeloma attends a cardiology clinic complaining of orthopnea, paroxysmal nocturnal dyspnea and bilateral leg swelling. On examination it is noticed that she has a large tongue, and her jugular venous pressure (JVP) rises on inspiration. Her echocardiogram reported her myocardium as having a 'sparkling appearance'. What is the underlying cause of this woman's breathlessness and ankle swelling?

A. Acromegaly
B. Acute kidney injury
C. Anaemia
D. Restrictive cardiomyopathy
E. Hypercalcaemia

1

3. A 52-year-old woman presents to the Accident and Emergency (A&E) department with crushing central chest pain. On examination cannon A waves can be seen when looking at the patient's jugular venous prssue (JVP) and she is bradycardic. An electrocardiogram (ECG) is performed. Which leads are most likely to show ST elevation?

A. II, III, aVF
B. V_1, V_2
C. V_3, V_4
D. V_5, V_6, I, aVL
E. Diffuse ST elevation throughout

4. A 24-year-old man attends a routine check up when it is noticed that his ECG shows a right bundle branch block pattern and ST elevation in leads V_1, V_2, and V_3. He doesn't report any chest pain or dyspnea, but has had two previous episodes of unexplained syncope. What is the underlying diagnosis?

A. Silent right-sided myocardial infarction
B. Tetralogy of Fallot
C. Brugada syndrome
D. Ventricular aneurysm
E. Myocarditis

5. A 45-year-old Afro-Caribbean male presents to the Accident and Emergency (A&E) department with a severe headache, whilst in A&E he loses conciseness and has a seizure lasting 3 minutes. His blood pressure is 220/130 mmHg and he has bilateral papilloedema on fundoscopy. Which of the following drugs is contraindicated in his immediate management?

A. Intravenous Furosemide
B. Intravenous labetalol
C. Intravenous sodium nitroprusside
D. Intravenous sodium thiosulfate
E. Sublingual nifedipine

6. A 28-year-old pregnant woman who recently started a new medication to treat hypertension develops palpitations and chest pain. On review of her blood tests her general practitioner notices she is anaemic and has a raised reticulocyte count. Which of the following medications should now be used to control her blood pressure?

A. Felodipine
B. Methyldopa
C. Atenolol
D. Labetalol
E. Captopril

7. A 75-year-old woman being treated for atrial fibrillation is reviewed in a cardiology outpatient clinic. She is currently on bisoprolol, ramipril and digoxin. A recent echocardiogram revealed systolic dysfunction and an ejection fraction of 35%. A new drug is added to her current medication to improve her prognosis. A week later she presents to the Accident and Emergency (A&E) department with xanthopsia, nausea, vomiting and confusion. Which of the following drugs did the cardiologist add?

A. Hydralazine
B. Verapamil
C. Indapamide
D. Amiloride
E. Spironolactone

8. A 30-year-old woman is brought into the Accident and Emergency (A&E) department with an ST-elevation myocardial infarction. She is immediately given aspirin, clopidogrel, morphine, metoclopramide and two puffs from a glyceryl trinitrate spray. She is immediately taken to the catheterisation laboratory for emergency intervention. A few hours later she develops diplopia, uncontrolled rotation of her eyeballs and severe jaw clenching. Which of the following drugs can be used to treat her symptoms?

A. Naloxone
B. Diazepam
C. Bromocriptine
D. Procyclidine
E. Baclofen

9. A 45-year-old woman with known systemic lupus erythematosus (SLE) presents to clinic complaining of central crushing chest pain that radiates to her left arm. It is only brought on by exertion, relieved by rest and not associated with vomiting. On taking a full history it became apparent that she experiences extreme pain in her fingers when it is cold. She describes them changing colour from white to blue, and then red. Which of the following drugs should she be used to treat her chest pain?

A. Aspirin
B. Propranolol
C. Nifedipine
D. Diltiazem
E. Simvastatin

10. A 67-year-old man with a prolonged history of intermittent haemoptysis, and dyspnea presents following a bout of dizziness and palpitations, which started only 2 days ago. He doesn't report any chest pain and his only significant past medical history is that he had rheumatic fever as a child, and he has never smoked. What is the underlying diagnosis?

A. Aortic stenosis
B. Lung cancer
C. Mitral stenosis
D. Pulmonary embolism
E. Infective endocarditis

11. A 54-year-old woman with a previous history of migraines is prescribed propranolol as prophylaxis. Following her first dose of propranolol she experiences central crushing chest pain. An electrocardiogram (ECG) shows ST elevation. Which of the following best describes the underlying pathology?

A. Asthma
B. Atheromatous plaque rupture
C. Brugada syndrome
D. Phaeochromocytoma
E. Prinzmetal's angina

12. A 22-year-old female presents with sharp central chest pain. This is worsened by inspiration and lying flat, but improves on sitting forward. An electrocardiogram (ECG) is performed. Which of the following is most likely to be seen?

A. Widespread ST elevation
B. Widespread ST depression
C. Shortened PR interval
D. J waves
E. U waves

13. Four weeks after a heart attack a patient attends a clinic for a routine check up. His electrocardiogram (ECG) shows persistent ST elevation and an echocardiogram reveals formation of a mural thrombus. What is the underling diagnosis?

A. Dressler's syndrome
B. Ventricular septal defect (VSD)
C. Left ventricular aneurysm
D. Unstable angina
E. Mitral regurgitation

14. A 14-year-old boy with a history of cystic fibrosis is admitted to hospital with a pseudomonal infection. Three days into his treatment he develops a broad complex tachycardia. Which of the following drugs has been used to treat his infection?

A. Piperacillin/tazobactam
B. Ceftazidime
C. Ciprofloxacin
D. Clarithromycin
E. Gentamicin

15. A 34-year-old Afro-Caribbean woman presents to clinic with increasing fatigue. She has symmetrical joint pain in her hands, alopecia and two painless mouth ulcers. On examination she is apyrexial but is found to have a collapsing pulse. What is the underlying cause of her aortic regurgitation?

A. Syphilitic aortitis
B. Psoriatic arthropathy
C. Infective endocarditis
D. Reiter's syndrome
E. Libman-Sacks endocarditis

16. Which of the following is most consistent with a diagnosis of aortic regurgitation?

A. Bounding pulse
B. Raised jugular venous pressure (JVP)
C. Narrow pulse pressure
D. Head nodding with every heartbeat
E. Loud A_2

17. A gentleman with atrial fibrillation and stable angina is referred to the cardiology clinic, because he is reporting chest pain on exertion despite already being treated with bisoprolol, amlodipine and warfarin. Which of the following medications could be added to improve his symptoms?

A. Ivabradine
B. Isosorbide mononitrate
C. Clopidogrel
D. Candesartan
E. Verapamil

18. A young boy reports recurrent episodes of palpations and dizziness. A resting electrocardiogram (ECG) shows a PR interval of 80ms, a delta wave and a broad QRS complex of 130ms. Which of the following is the definitive treatment for this patients underlying condition?

A. Implantation of an implantable cardioverter-defibrillator (ICD)
B. Radiofrequency ablation of the bundle of Kent
C. Atrioventricular node ablation and implantation of a permanent pacemaker
D. Oral verapamil
E. Intravenous adenosine

19. A 70-year-old man with a background of diabetes, hypertension and peripheral vascular disease presents with chest pain at rest. The pain is central and radiates to his left arm. He has had episodes of chest pain for the last 4 weeks and they have become more frequent and prolonged in nature. His initial blood tests do not demonstrate a rise in troponin T. Which of the following is the most appropriate next step in this patient's managment?

A. Dobutamine stress echocardiogram
B. CT coronary angiogram
C. Myocardial perfusion scintigraphy (MPS)
D. Cardiac magnetic resonance imaging (MRI)
E. Coronary angiogram +/- percutaneous coronary intervention

20. A 13-month-old child presents to hospital with breathlessness. On examination he is found to be apyrexial, have finger clubbing, a left parasternal heave and a harsh pan systolic murmur. A chest X-ray shows a boot shaped heart. Which of the following is the most likely diagnosis?

A. Tetralogy of Fallot
B. Ventricular septal defect
C. Atrial septal defect
D. Infective endocarditis
E. Atrial myxoma

21. Which of the following is not a cause of a dilated cardiomyopathy?

A. Hyperthyroidism
B. Hypothyroidism
C. Coxsackie B virus myocarditis
D. Becker's muscular dystrophy
E. Cisplatin therapy

22. A patient presents to his general practice (GP) with a 3-week history of a persistent dry cough, facial flushing and wheeze. On examination a pan systolic murmur can be heard. It is loudest on inspiration at the left lower sternal edge. Which of the following set of investigations should be used to confirm the underlying diagnosis?

A. Blood cultures and an echocardiogram
B. DNAse O titre and an echocardiogram
C. Urinary metadrenaline and normetadrenaline
D. Urinary 5-hydroxyindoleacetic acid
E. Electrocardiogram (ECG) and troponin T

23. A 24-year-old cocaine user presents to the Accident and Emergency (A&E) department with chest pain that radiates towards his back. On examination it is noticed that his left pupil is constricted and there is partial ptosis of the left eyelid. What is the most likely diagnosis?

A. Myocardial infarction
B. Myocarditis
C. Aortic dissection
D. Oesophageal spasm
E. Gastro-oesophageal reflux disease

24. A patient presents to the Accident and Emergency (A&E) department with central crushing chest pain and two episodes of vomiting. On examination the patient is hypotensive and has a raised jugular venous pressure (JVP), but on auscultation the lung bases are clear. An electrocardiogram (ECG) shows ST elevation in leads II, III, aVF and also in V_1 and V_2. Which of the following is the most appropriate next step in this patient's management?

A. Dobutamine infusion
B. 2 puffs of glyceryl trinitrate (GTN) spray and 10 mg of intravenous morphine
C. 10 mg of intravenous metoclopramide
D. 500 mls of intravenous 0.9% saline
E. 15 L of oxygen via a reservoir mask

25. A gentleman is diagnosed with a non-ST elevation myocardial infarction over night. He is deemed to be a low risk patient and therefore will wait till the next day for his coronary angiogram. He has already been given aspirin and ticagrelor. Which of the following medications should he be given while waiting for a coronary angiogram?

A. Clopidogrel
B. Warfarin
C. Alteplase
D. Fondaparinux
E. Ramipril

26. An 80-year-old female attends a general practice (GP) appointment complaining of paroxysmal nocturnal dyspnea and orthopnea. On examination she is found to have a raised jugular venous pressure (JVP), bilateral ankle swelling and fine inspiratory crepitations. She is prescribed furosemide and sent home, but unfortunately passes away two days later. Which of the following is likely to be found in the lungs during a post-mortem?

A. Red hepatisation
B. Hyaline membrane thickening
C. Fibrin clot formation
D. Interstitial infiltration by lymphocytes
E. Haemosiderin laden macrophages

27. A 35-year-old lady is admitted to hospital two weeks after an aortic valve replacement with a fever of 39 degrees Celsius. Blood cultures are taken from three different sites. The results of the blood cultures will not be available for 48 hours. Which of the following antibiotic regimes should be commenced?

A. Benzylpenicillin and gentamicin
B. Flucloxacillin and gentamicin
C. Amoxicillin and gentamicin
D. Vancomycin and gentamicin
E. Meropenem and gentamicin

28. A 65-year-old lady attends her general practice (GP) for a review. On examination it is found that she has an irregularly irregular pulse at a rate of 70 bpm. She has not complained of any dyspnea, palpitations, chest pain or ankle swelling. Which of the following is the best management option?

A. Review in 6 months
B. Anticoagulate with clopidogrel
C. Anticoagulate with warfarin
D. Rhythm control with amiodarone
E. Refer to a cardiologist

29. A 65-year-old man with severe heart failure is suffering from uncomfortable leg swelling. On examination he is found to have bilateral pitting oedema 5 cm above his knees. He currently takes bisoprolol, captopril, spironolactone and furosemide all at their maximum daily dosage. His renal function is good. Which of the following drugs would be most appropriate to help improve his symptoms?

A. Candesartan
B. Digoxin
C. Acetazolamide
D. Metolazone
E. Mannitol

30. A 30-year-old asthmatic presents to the Accident and Emergency (A&E) department with a one hour history of palpitations and crushing chest pain. She is diagnosed with a supraventricular tachycardia. Which of the following is the most appropriate form of treatment for this patient?

A. Intravenous adenosine
B. Intravenous metoprolol
C. Intravenous verapamil
D. Synchronized direct current (DC) cardioversion
E. Unsynchronized direct current (DC) cardioversion

31. A 30-year-old female with a history of depression presents complaining of a blurred vision, dry eyes and a dry mouth. On examination she is found to have a dull suprapubic mass. Her electrocardiogram (ECG) shows that she is tachycardic, with a widened QRS complex and a prolonged QTc. Her arterial blood gas shows a metabolic acidosis with a raised anion gap. Which of the following treatment regimes should be started first?

A. Intravenous calcium gluconate
B. Intravenous insulin and 50% dextrose
C. Intravenous sodium bicarbonate
D. Intravenous digibind
E. Haemodialysis

Cardiology Answers

1. C
Constrictive pericarditis

This man has presented with signs of heart failure, and on examination Kussmaul's sign can be seen (which is a rise in the JVP on inspiration). Constrictive pericarditis can be caused by tuberculosis, but is most commonly idiopathic. Constrictive pericarditis is a cause of diastolic heart failure as it affects the filling of the heart. It often presents with signs of right-sided heart failure first, followed by congestive cardiac failure.

The only other option here that can cause Kussmaul's sign is cardiac tamponade, but this is less likely because in tamponade the patient would be hypotensive, tachycardic, have muffled heart sounds and be very unwell. The combination of a falling blood pressure, rising JVP and quiet heart sounds (which can occur in cardiac tamponade) is known as Beck's triad.

Tricuspid regurgitation would cause a large V wave in the JVP. It also causes a pan-systolic murmur heard loudest at the left parasternal edge on expiration, with no radiation. Other signs on examination would include pulsatile hepatomegaly and bilateral ankle swelling.

Pulmonary hypertension could also cause a raised JVP, hepatomegaly and ankle swelling if it progresses to cause cor pulmonale (right ventricular failure as a result of pulmonary hypertension). It can also cause a loud P2 and parasternal heave due to right ventricular hypertrophy.

Dilated cardiomyopathy is a cause of systolic heart failure and would also cause all the signs of congestive cardiac failure. There are many causes of dilated cardiomyopathy; infectious causes would include a viral myocarditis and Chagas disease.

2. D
Restrictive cardiomyopathy

This woman has a developed congestive heart failure. She has developed orthopnea and paroxysmal nocturnal dyspnea which are signs of left sided heart failure, and bilateral ankle swelling and a raised JVP, which are signs of right sided heart failure.

The underlying cause of her heart failure is a restrictive cardiomyopathy, secondary to her multiple myeloma, which is caused by deposition of AL amyloid in the myocardium. This presents very similarly to constrictive pericarditis, with Kussmaul's sign and signs of right-sided heart failure. Restrictive cardiomyopathy due to amyloidosis is thought to give a 'sparkling' appearance on the echocardiogram.

The macroglossia seen is also due to AL amyloid deposition. Macroglossia can occur in acromegaly but acromegaly would cause a dilated cardiomyopathy, which would not cause Kussmaul's sign.

The only other cause of heart failure listed is anaemia, and this would cause a high output heart failure.

Renal failure, anaemia and hypercalcaemia are all other features of multiple myeloma.

3. A
II, III, aVF

This patient has had an inferior infarct involving the right coronary artery. This supplies the atrioventricular (AV) node, and the infarct has caused complete heart block, resulting in cannon A waves and bradycardia. Cannon A waves can be seen whenever the right atrium contracts against a closed tricuspid valve, such as in complete heart block, ventricular ectopics, ventricular arrhythmias and single chamber ventricular pacing.

V_1 and V_2 ST elevation would occur in a septal infarction. V_3 and V_4 ST elevation would occur in an anterior infarction. An anterior infarct can also cause complete heart block in some cases, where the left anterior descending artery supplies the AV node. This is a rare varient, and far less common. V_5, V_6, I and aVL ST elevation would occur in a lateral myocardial infarction.

Diffuse ST elevation can be seen in pericarditis and often has a saddle shape appearance. It doesn't follow the pattern of the coronary blood supply and can be accompanied by PR interval depression.

4. C
Brugada syndrome

Right bundle branch block pattern and ST elevation in leads V_1, V_2, and V_3 are a classic presentation of Brugada syndrome. This condition most commonly has an autosomal dominant inheritance pattern and predisposes patients to developing fatal arrhythmias. It often has a strong family history of unexplained syncope and sudden unexplained death. It is treated with an implantable cardiac defibrillator (ICD).

A right-sided myocardial infarction often occurs in conjunction with an inferior myocardial infarction, due to both areas being supplied by the right coronary artery. An old infarction may show Q-waves in the inferior leads. This patient is too young to have developed have had an old myocardial infarction.

Tetralogy of Fallot is a congenital cyanotic heart condition, which comprises of a ventricular septal defect, overriding aorta, pulmonary stenosis and right ventricular hypertrophy. The combination causes a right to left shunt. It presents early in life with poor growth and episodes of cyanosis.

A ventricular aneurysm occurs 4–6 weeks after a myocardial infarction due to weakening of the myocardium. It presents with persistent ST elevation. It can also lead to systemic emboli.

Myocarditis is caused by inflammation of the cardiac muscle often as a result of a viral infection. It presents with fever and cardiac chest pain. The ECG may show non-specific ST changes, arrhythmias and a transient atrioventricular (AV) block.

5. E
Sublingual nifedipine

This patient has presented with malignant hypertension, and because of his headache and seizure he is likely to have developed an encephalopathy. The aim of treatment in this case is to reduce the diastolic blood pressure to less than 110 mmHg over the next 4 hours. This is started by giving furosemide (loop diuretic which causes venodilation) followed by either labetalol (a beta-blocker) or sodium nitroprusside. Sodium nitroprusside is a potent vasodilator that is broken down into nitric oxide. If high doses are given, it must be given in conjunction with sodium thiosulfate to reduce the risk of cyanide poisoning.

Nifedipine is a dihydropyridine calcium channel blocker. It should never be given in malignant hypertension (especially in its sub-lingual form), as it can reduce the blood pressure too rapidly and thus cause an ischaemic stroke, due to hypoperfusion.

6. D
Labetalol

This patient was being treated with methyldopa for her hypertension. However this caused a haemolytic anaemia, which lead to symptoms of chest pain and palpitations. The drug should therefore be discontinued and she should be treated with labetalol, which is another antihypertensive that is safe to use in pregnancy.

The only antihypertensive drugs that are deemed safe to use in pregnancy are labetalol, nifedipine, methyldopa and hydralazine. All others are seen as unsafe or have relative contraindications.

7. E
Spironolactone

This woman has developed digoxin toxicity. Digoxin inhibits the sodium/potassium pump in the myocardium, thus causing increased intracellular calcium. This results in a positive ionotropic effect and reduced heart rate. It is used to treat heart failure and atrial fibrillation.

Digoxin toxicity presents with nausea, vomiting, confusion, arrhythmias and xanthopsia. It can be due to electrolyte imbalances such as hypokalaemia, hypomagnesaemia and hypercalcaemia. Other precipitants of toxicity include hypothyroidism, hypoalbuminaemia, and a long list of medications.

Out of the following drugs indapamide is the only drug that causes hypokalaemia. However it is a thiazide-like diuretic used to treat hypertension and is therefore not indicated in this patient. Spironolactone can cause toxicity because despite it being a potassium sparing diuretic, it also competes for the same receptor as digoxin for excretion, thus causing levels to rise. Spironolactone is the most likely drug to be added in this scenario, because along with bisoprolol and ramipril, it improves prognosis in heart failure patients.

Other drugs that can cause digoxin toxicity include amiodarone, verapamil and diltiazem. Verapamil is listed here, but would not have been prescribed in this patient; firstly because it has a negative inotropic effect and therefore is contraindicated in heart failure, and secondly because she is already taking a beta-blocker. Non-dihydropyridine calcium channel blockers, such as verapamil, shouldn't be prescribed in conduction with beta-blockers because both classes of drug act on the atrioventricular (AV) node, and if prescribed together can cause complete heart block.

Hydralazine is an antihypertensive drug used in hypertension resistant to other first line drugs. It binds to and activates potassium channels on the smooth muscle cells and causes vasodilation. It can be used in conjunction with isosorbide dinitrate to treat congestive cardiac failure in Afro-Caribbean patients who are resistant to other medications.

8. D
Procyclidine

This patient has developed an oculogyric crisis, which is a side effect of metoclopramide. Metoclopramide is an antiemetic, which is a dopamine D2-receptor antagonist and is also a pro-kinetic agent. It has the same mechanism as domperidone, however domperidone cannot cross the blood brain barrier and therefore doesn't cause an oculogyric crisis. Domperidone does however cause long QT syndrome and therefore should be avoided in patients who are at risk of this, such as those with a history of ischaemic heart disease.

An oculogyric crisis presents with restlessness, diplopia, uncontrolled upward deviation of the eyes and a fixed stare. It can also result from use of antipsychotic drugs, due to their D2-antagonistic properties. An oculogyric crisis can be treated by use of the anticholinergic drug procyclidine.

Naloxone is an opiate receptor antagonist, which is given in opiate overdoses.

Diazepam is a benzodiazepine with a long half-life and can be used as an anxiolytic, to treated seizures and as a muscle relaxant.

Bromocriptine is a dopamine receptor agonist, which is used to treat microprolactinomas and Parkinson's disease.

Baclofen is a GABA B receptor agonist and is used as a muscle relaxant.

9. D
Diltiazem

This patient has stable angina. Normally the first line treatment for this would be to give a beta-blocker. However this patient also has severe Raynaud's disease and therefore beta-blockers are contraindicated. Instead a non-dihydropyridine calcium channel blocker should be used such as diltiazem or verapamil. These act on the atrioventricular (AV) node to control heart rate and thus provide symptomatic relief. Furthermore propranolol is not cardio-selective and acts all over the body, therefore is not commonly used to treat angina.

Aspirin and simvastatin are likely to be prescribed to reduce the risk of a future myocardial infarction, but do not provide symptomatic relief.

Nifedipine is a dihydropyridine calcium channel blocker, which causes vasodilation. It is used to treat Raynaud's phenomenon, hypertension and also as a second line drug in angina.

10. C
Mitral stenosis

Rheumatic fever is caused by a Streptococcus pyogenes infection of the throat. It leads to autoantibodies being created against the heart valves and can cause both mitral and aortic stenosis.

This patient has underlying mitral stenosis. It causes left atrial hypertrophy and leads to atrial fibrillation. This patient has developed atrial fibrillation, hence the palpitations and dizziness. Mitral stenosis is also a cause of haemoptysis.

Aortic stenosis is often asymptomatic, but can cause angina, dyspnea and syncope.

Lung cancer can also cause haemoptysis and dyspnea but doesn't link in with the history of rheumatic fever.

Pulmonary embolism is more likely to have a sudden onset of symptoms and often would cause chest pain.

Infective endocarditis should always be considered in patients with a fever and a new murmur. This patient would be at risk of infective endocarditis because he already has valvular disease, however none of the features suggestive of infective endocarditis have been described.

11. E
Prinzmetal's angina

This is also known as vasospasm angina, and is where chest pain is caused by spasm of the coronary arteries. It is sometimes linked to other vasospasm disorders such as Raynaud's syndrome and migraines. Beta-blockers and aspirin are known to worsen the vasospasm and are therefore contraindicated. Treatment is often with nitrates and calcium channel blockers.

Brugada syndrome is an autosomal dominant condition that predisposes patients to developing fatal arrhythmias. It often has a strong family history of unexplained syncope and sudden unexplained death. An ECG would show right bundle branch block pattern and ST elevation in leads V_1, V_2, and V_3. Also it doesn't cause chest pain.

Atheromatous plaque rupture would present with chest pain and ST elevation in the form of a ST elevation myocardial infarction, however it wouldn't be precipitated by a beta-blockers. Beta-blockers are now used as secondary prevention, and have a cardio-protective effect, by preventing excessive strain on the myocardium.

Phaeochromocytoma is a carcinoma of the adrenal medulla, which results in overproduction of catecholamines. Symptoms would include palpitations, sweating, anxiety and headaches. Treatment is to give phenoxybenzamine (alpha-blocker) followed by propranolol (beta-blocker). Definitive treatment is surgery. If propranolol is given first it causes a crisis due to unopposed alpha-adrenergic stimulation.

Beta-blockers, non-steroidal anti-inflammatory drugs (NSAIDs) and aspirin can worsen asthma. Therefore an attack could be triggered by propranolol. It would present with chest tightness, shortness of breath and cough. However it wouldn't cause ST elevation on an ECG, and new onset asthma in a 54-year-old is also unlikely.

12. B
Widespread ST elevation

This patient has pericarditis. This is inflammation of the pericardial lining of the heart. It can be idiopathic or secondary due to infections (such as coxsackie B virus, Epstein-Barr virus (EBV), mumps), myocardial infarction, Dressler's syndrome, uraemia or autoimmune conditions (rheumatoid arthritis, systemic lupus erythematosus (SLE), sarcoidosis). It classically causes pleuritic chest pain that is worse on lying flat and on inspiration, and relieved by leaning forward. An ECG shows widespread saddle shaped ST elevation, which doesn't adhere to any vascular territory.

Widespread ST depression can occur in patients who are on digoxin and this classically causes reverse tick ST depression. ST depression can occur in acute coronary syndrome, but is more likely to adhere to a vascular territory.

A shortened PR interval occurs where there is an accessory pathway connecting the atria and ventricles, such as in Wolff-Parkinson-White syndrome, where this pathway is known as the bundle of Kent.

J waves occur just after the QRS complex and are seen in hypothermia. Other features of hypothermia include bradycardia, prolonged PR interval and a prolonged QT interval.

U waves occur in hypokalaemia. Other features of hypokalaemia include prolonged PR interval, flattened or inverted T-waves and a prolonged QT interval.

13. C
Left ventricular aneurysm

This can occur 4-6 weeks after a myocardial infarction, due to weakening of the myocardium and formation of scar tissue. It can present with persistent ST elevation, angina and ventricular arrhythmias. Due to dysfunction of the ventricular wall there is stasis of blood and it can cause formation of a mural thrombus. This patient requires surgery to correct the aneurysm and also anticoagulation to prevent an embolic stroke. This is the only cause listed that would cause a mural thrombus to form.

Dressler's syndrome develops 1–3 weeks after a myocardial infarction and is due to the myocardial injury stimulating production of antibodies against the myocardium. This leads to pericardial inflammation and presents with fever, pleuritic chest pain, and it can progress to a pericardial effusion. The ECG may show widespread saddle shaped ST elevation as a result of the pericarditis.

A ventricular septal defect can occur in the first 4–7 days after a myocardial infarction and is due to rupture of the septum as a result of ischaemic damage. It presents with cardiac failure and a pan-systolic murmur.

Mitral regurgitation occurs within the first 10 days after a myocardial infarction and is due to either due to papillary muscle or chordae tendineae rupture. It also presents with cardiac failure and a pan-systolic murmur.

Unstable angina would present with episodes of central crushing chest pain at rest. The ECG may show ST depression during these episodes.

14. C
Ciprofloxacin

Ciprofloxacin is a quinolone and acts by inhibition of DNA gyrase. It is the only oral antibiotic that can be used to treat a pseudomonal infection. Intravenous antibiotics with anti-pseudomonal properties include: gentamicin, piperacillin/tazobactam, meropenem and ceftazidine.

Side effects of ciprofloxacin include lowering the seizure threshold, Achilles tendon rupture and importantly for this question, drug induced long QT syndrome.

Long QT syndrome can lead to torsades de pointes, which is a polymorphic ventricular tachycardia. Long QT can be caused by electrolyte imbalances (hypokalaemia, hypomagnesaemia and hypocalcaemia), hypothermia and also genetic conditions (Romano-Ward and Jervell and Lange-Nielsen syndrome). Other drug causes include anti-arrythmics (class I and class III), antibiotics (macrolides and quinolones), antipsychotics and antidepressants (tricyclics and citalopram).

The only other drug listed here that causes long QT is clarithromycin, but this doesn't work against pseudomonas and therefore wouldn't have been used.

15. E
Libman-Sacks endocarditis

This patient has got underlying systemic lupus erythematosus (SLE) (hence the small joint polyarthritis, mouth ulcers and alopecia). She has developed Libman-Sacks endocarditis. This is where sterile destructive vegetations form on the heart valves and cause scarring and regurgitation murmurs. In this case it has caused aortic regurgitation. All the other options can cause aortic regurgitation but are less likely due to the clinical picture.

Syphilitic aortitis takes many years to develop. It occurs as part of quaternary syphilis and can also cause thoracic aortic aneurysms. It would often be accompanied by tabes dorsalis and dementia as a result of neuro-syphilis.

Psoriatic arthropathy is a seronegative arthopathy and would often present with a psoriatic rash (salmon pink plaques on the extensor surfaces with a silvery scale). It has many joint patterns but can also cause a symmetrical polyarthritis.

Reiter's syndrome is a form of reactive arthritis, which presents with a triad of urethritis, arthritis and conjunctivitis. This often follows a sexually transmitted infection (STI) or dysentery.

Infective endocarditis would present with a fever and a new murmur. However this patient is apyrexial so this is less likely.

16. D
Head nodding with every heart beat

This is known as De Musset's sign, and can occur in severe aortic regurgitation. Aortic regurgitation also causes a wide pulse pressure, collapsing pulse and a soft A2. Other signs of aortic regurgitation include the following:

Quincke's sign: capillary pulsations in the nail beds
Corrigan's sign: carotid pulsation
Traube's sign: a pistol shot sound heard over the femoral arteries

A Bounding pulse can be found in sepsis, liver failure and carbon dioxide retention.

Raised JVP can be due to right ventricular failure, liver failure, renal failure, or fluid overload.

Narrow pulse pressure can be seen in aortic stenosis, constrictive pericarditis and cardiac tamponade.

A loud A2 could be due to systemic hypertension or a metallic sounding A2 would occur following a valve replacement.

17. D
Isosorbide mononitrate

This gentleman has stable angina and is already being treated with a beta-blocker (which is first line treatment) and a calcium-channel blocker. Despite this he is symptomatic, and therefore a third agent needs to be initiated. Long acting nitrates (such as isosorbide mononitrate) cause vasodilation and improve blood flow through the coronary arteries. They are a useful adjunct in patients who are already on first line therapy.

Ivabradine acts on the I_f channel in the sinoatrial node to reduce the heart rate. It can be used in patients with angina, which is not adequately controlled by beta-blockers, but is only effective in those who are in sinus rhythm, and wouldn't work in atrial fibrillation.

Clopidogrel is an antiplatelet medication used following percutaneous coronary intervention (PCI). This is not indicated unless the patient has undergone PCI. Furthermore this gentleman is already on warfarin and clopidogrel would increase his risk of bleeding without any prognostic or symptomatic benefit.

Candesartan is an angiotensin II receptor blocker, used in patients with hypertension or heart failure who do not tolerate angiotensin converting enzyme (ACE) inhibitors. It would not reduce symptoms in patients with angina.

Verapamil is a non-dihydropyridine calcium channel blocker, which can be used as first line treatment for angina or rate control in atrial fibrillation, in patients who do not tolerate beta-blockers. However it should not be used in conjunction with beta-blockers as the combination can lead to heart block.

18. C
Radiofrequency ablation of the bundle of Kent

This patient has Wolff-Parkinson-White syndrome, which is where an accessory pathway (known as the bundle of Kent) connects the atria and the ventricles. This pathway allows electrical activity to bypass the atrioventricular (AV) node and can result in tachyarrhythmias. It is diagnosed on the basis of an ECG showing a shortened PR interval (<120 ms), a delta wave (which is a slurred upstroke in the QRS complex), and a broad QRS complex (>120 ms). The definitive treatment is radiofrequency ablation of the bundle of Kent.

Drugs that act to block the AV node (such as verapamil and adenosine) are contraindicated because by blocking the heart's normal electrical pathway they can exacerbate the excitation through the bundle of Kent, leading to potentially dangerous arrhythmias.

Implantation of an implantable cardioverter-defibrillator (ICD) would be used to treat patients who have had previous episodes of ventricular tachycardia or ventricular fibrillation, such as in a patient with ischaemic heart disease or Brugada syndrome.

AV node ablation and implantation of a permanent pacemaker is the last line treatment for patients with atrial fibrillation who have been resistant to both pharmacological therapy and direct current (DC) cardioversion.

19. E
Coronary angiogram +/- percutaneous coronary intervention

This gentleman has presented with crescendo angina, which is unstable angina that is worsening. It is characterised by episodes of chest pain become more frequent, severe or prolonged. The reason for this is that he has cardiac chest pain, which is occurring at rest, but without any rise in his troponin. This gentleman is at a high risk of atherosclerotic plaque rupture leading to a myocardial infarction and therefore needs an urgent coronary angiogram. If there is an area of significant stenosis this will require percutaneous coronary intervention.

A CT coronary angiogram is a non-invasive imaging tool that allows imaging of the coronary arteries. It is often used in patients who are at a lower risk of coronary artery disease.

Cardiac magnetic resonance imaging is useful at assessing the viability of the myocardium. It is used in the diagnosis of myocarditis.

Dobutamine stress echocardiogram and myocardial perfusion scintigraphy are both imaging techniques used to assess the function of the heart muscle, and can be used to plan coronary angioplasty in patients with coronary artery disease by assessing the viability of the muscle. However these are used to plan elective procedures and are not used in high-risk patients, like this gentleman.

20. A
Tetralogy of Fallot

Tetralogy of Fallot is a congenital heart defect, which presents with a ventricular septal defect (hence the pan systolic murmur), pulmonary stenosis, right ventricular hypertrophy (hence the left parasternal heave) and the aorta overriding the ventricular septal defect. The combination of both pulmonary stenosis and a ventricular septal defect leads to a right to left shunt and the blood bypassing the lungs. Cyanotic congenital heart disease is another cause of clubbing. The boot shapped heart is characteristic of Tetralogy of Fallot.

Both a large ventricular septal defect and a large atrial septal defect can lead to cyanosis. This is by causing Eisenmenger's syndrome, which is where there is originally a left to right shunt due to the heart defect. This causes pulmonary hypertension, right ventricular hypertrophy and shunt reversal to a right to left shunt. This is less likely due to the boot shaped heart, and because Eisenmenger's syndrome takes longer to develop.

Infective endocarditis is unlikely as the patient is apyrexial.

An atrial myxoma is a benign tumour of the heart, and is the most common type of primary heart tumour. It often forms in the atria. It can present similarly to infective endocarditis and a 'tumour plop' may also be heard on auscultation.

21. E
Cisplatin

Cisplatin is a chemotherapeutic drug, which can cause both nephrotoxicity and ototoxicity. Anthracycline chemotheraptic drugs such as doxorubicin can cause dilated cardiomyopathy. Other causes include both hyper and hypothyroidism, post-viral myocarditis, alcohol, haemochromatosis, sacroidosis and congenital X-linked defects in the dystrophin gene such as in Becker's and Duchenne's muscular dystrophy. These all lead to an intrinsic myocardial abnormality. Causes of secondary/indirect myocardial dysfunction causing a dilated heart are ischaemic heart disease, valvular heart disease, and hypertension. Hyperthyroidism can also cause a high output heart failure.

22. D
Urinary 5-hydroxyindoleacetic acid

This patient has carcinoid syndrome, which is caused by a neuroendocrine tumour producing serotonin. It presents with a cough, flushing, headaches, wheeze and diarrhoea. It also affects the heart causing tricuspid regurgitation and pulmonary stenosis. The diagnosis can be made by testing for urinary 5-hydroxyindoleacetic acid, which is a serotonin metabolite. Carcinoid tumours most commonly occur in the bowel, but would only present with symptoms once they have metastasized to the liver. Before then the liver metabolises any serotonin produced. Once metastasis occurs it skips the first pass metabolism. Other sites for primaries include the lungs, and these tumours would cause symptoms straight away, as there is no first pass metabolism. Medical treatment is by use of octeotride (a somatostatin analogue) and definitive treatment is surgical resection.

Blood cultures and an echocardiogram can be used to diagnose bacterial endocarditis. This patient does have a new murmur, which would make us suspect infective endocarditis however the cough, wheeze and facial flushing point towards carcinoid syndrome.

DNAse O titre and anti-streptolysin O titre can be used to diagnose rheumatic fever. This is unlikely in this patient as there is no complaint of a sore throat or rash (such as scarlet fever or erythema marginatum). Also rheumatic fever is more likely to affect the left side of the heart and cause mitral and aortic stenosis.

Urinary metadrenaline and normetadrenaline levels are used to diagnose a phaeochromocytoma. This is likely to cause headaches, palpitations, sweating and spontaneous rises in blood pressure.

ECG and troponin T (a cardiac enzyme) would be used if an acute myocardial infarction were suspected. This is extremely unlikely in this patient, as there is no report of chest pain.

23. C
Aortic dissection

This patient has presented with aortic dissection, which is a tear of the tunica intima of the aorta, allowing blood to flow through the layers of the aorta. Classically it presents with severe tearing chest pain that radiates to the back. If the tear extends upwards it can also involve the carotid arteries, thus disrupting the sympathetic nerves and causing Horner's syndrome; which is evident in this patient who has a constricted pupil and ptosis, other features would include enophthalmos and anhidrosis. If the tear occurs downwards it can result in aortic regurgitation, and if it affects the coronary arteries can cause a myocardial infarction. Type A involves the ascending aorta and these patients must be considered for surgery, while type B doesn't involve the ascending aorta and may be managed medically. Cocaine use is also a risk factor for aortic dissection; other risk factors include hypertension, connective tissue disorders, bicuspid aortic valve, and chest trauma.

Myocardial infarction would cause central crushing chest pain radiating to the neck and left arm. It is often associated with nausea, vomiting and sweating. Cocaine use is also a risk factor for myocardial infarction.

Myocarditis is likely to cause a fever and central chest pain. It is often preceded by flu like symptoms.

Oesophageal spasm can cause central cardiac sounding chest pain, but would also cause intermittent dysphagia.

Gastro-oesophageal reflux disease can cause a burning retrosternal chest pain. Out of all these conditions, aortic dissection is the only one that would be associated with Horner's syndrome.

24. D
500 mls of intravenous 0.9% saline

This patient has presented with an inferior myocardial infarction, as is evident by the ST elevation in leads II, III, and aVF. This patient also has had a right ventricular infarction. This can occur in up to 40% of patients with an inferior myocardial infarction due to the blood supply of the right coronary artery. It should also be suspected in any patient presenting with the triad of a raised JVP, hypotension and clear lungs. Further evidence of this is the ST elevation in lead V_1, which is the closest lead to the right ventricle. The first line treatment is fluid resuscitation, which aims to increase the right ventricular preload.

Dobutamine is an inotrope used in intensive care if all other measures have failed.

Nitrates are contraindicated in right ventricular infarctions, because the vasodilation leads to a reduced venous return and reduced preload. Therefore nitrites would cause profound hypotension.

Metoclopramide may be useful to prevent the vomiting induced by the myocardial infarction and is often given to with morphine, because opiates can cause nausea and vomiting. However it is not as important as intravenous fluids.

There is nothing to suggest this patient has desaturated and therefore oxygen is not necessary. Oxygen should only be given in an acute myocardial infarction if the oxygen saturations are below 94%, due to a fear of re-perfusion injury.

25. D
Fondaparinux

Patients who are diagnosed with a non-ST elevation myocardial infarction require percutaneous coronary intervention (PCI). However the urgency of this is determined by the individuals risk based on the GRACE score. If a patient's PCI is delayed then they are given either fondaparinux or low molecular weight heparin (often in the form of enoxaparin) while they wait for their procedure. Both of these drugs are factor Xa inhibitors and act to prevent further clot formation.

Patients awaiting PCI are started on dual antiplatelet agents, with aspirin and either clopidogrel or ticagrelor. Both clopidogrel and ticagrelor act on the $P2Y_{12}$ platelet receptor, and therefore are never prescribed together.

Warfarin is not indicated in acute coronary syndrome treatment. Its indications include: treatment of a deep vein thrombosis or pulmonary embolism, anticoagulation for a metallic heart valve and to prevent systemic emboli in atrial fibrillation.

Alteplase is an agent used for thrombolysis and would only be indicated in an ST elevation myocardial infarction where PCI is not available.

Ramipril is an angiotensin converting enzyme (ACE) inhibitor and is often initiated after PCI as it has cardio-protective properties. However it would not be started prior to an angiogram because it is nephrotoxic and may increase the chance of contrast-induced nephropathy.

26. E
Haemosiderin laden macrophages

This patient is in congestive cardiac failure and as a result has developed pulmonary oedema. High pulmonary blood pressure has resulted in red blood cells passing through the capillaries into the alveoli. Alveolar macrophages phagocytose these red blood cells and become engorged in haemosiderin. They are also known as heart failure cells. Haemosiderin laden macrophages are also found in areas of haemorrhage.

Red hepatisation occurs in pneumonia, and is where the blood vessels in the lung become more permeable, and red cells and neutrophils enter the lungs. This precedes grey hepatisation where the red cells are digested and the only remaining cells are the neutrophils.

Hyaline membrane thickening is found in acute respiratory distress syndrome (ARDS).

Fibrin clot formation can be found in a pulmonary embolism, or if there are multiple fibrin clots found all over the body then disseminated intravascular coagulation may be suspected.

Interstitital infiltration by lymphocytes can occur in a viral pneumonitis or can be found in idiopathic pulmonary fibrosis and autoimmune causes of pulmonary fibrosis such as sarcoidosis and systemic lupus erythematosus (SLE).

27. D
Vancomycin and gentamicin

This patient has had a recent valve replacement and therefore is at risk of infective endocarditis. Within 6 months of a valve replacement the most likely organisms would be Staphylococcus epidermis (also know as coagulase negative Staphylococcus) and methicillin-resistant Staphylococcus aureus (MRSA). The empirical treatment of choice for a prosthetic valve infective endocarditis within 6 months of surgery is vancomycin and gentamicin, because this will cover an MRSA infection.

Staphylococcus aureus infective endocarditis can also occur in intravenous drug users, and in these patients often affects the right side of the heart. Flucloxacillin and gentamicin can be used to treat these patients.

Pseudomonas bacteraemias can occur as a result of iatrogenic lines such as a central line. These infections can be difficult to treat and may require use of broad-spectrum antibiotics such as meropenem.

Viridians Streptococci are a common cause of infective endocarditis in native valves and classically occurs following dental procedures. This can be treated with benzylpenicillin and gentamicin. This combination is used as empirical treatment in patients who have not had a recent valve replacement.

Enterococcus infective endocarditis is associated with prolonged urinary tract infections, and gastrointestinal surgery. If grown in a blood culture it can be treated with amoxicillin and gentamicin.

28. C
Anticoagulate with warfarin

The main treatment for atrial fibrillation is comprised of rate control, rhythm control and anticoagulation to prevent stroke. The need for anticoagulation is calculated using the CHA_2DS_2-VASc score. If 2 or more then patients require anticoagulation. This patient scores 1 for being 65–74 years old and 1 for being female, and therefore requires anticoagulation.

Clopidogrel is not used for anticoagulation in atrial fibrillation. It is an antiplatelet agent used in secondary prevention of myocardial infarctions and ischaemic strokes.

Rate control with beta-blockers is preferred in elderly patients. Therefore in this patient amiodarone is not an appropriate option. Rhythm control may be preferred in young patients, who have reversible causes, and are symptomatic; or patients who are in congestive cardiac failure as it improves cardiac output.

29. D
Metolazone

Metolazone is a thiazide-like diuretic and therefore acts in the distal convoluted tubule by inhibiting the sodium chloride co-transporter. It is extremely potent and not used to treat hypertension, but instead used to offload fluid in heart failure. It would only be introduced if patients were already on high doses of a loop diuretic and potassium sparing diuretic. When using such a drug renal function must be monitored as it could cause dehydration and subsequent pre-renal failure.

Candesartan is an angiotensin II receptor blocker. It is used if angiotensin converting enzyme (ACE) inhibitors can't be tolerated. This patient is already on an ACE inhibitor and therefore it is not indicated.

Acetazolamide is a carbonic anhydrase inhibitor, which prevents bicarbonate reabsorption in the proximal convoluted tubule. It causes a metabolic acidosis with a normal anion gap. It can be used to treat idiopathic intracranial hypertension, acute angle glaucoma and as prophylaxis for altitude sickness.

Mannitol is an osmotic diuretic, which is used in patients with raised intracranial pressure.

Digoxin inhibits the sodium/potassium pump in the myocardium, thus causing increased intracellular calcium. This results in a positive ionotropic effect and reduced heart rate. It is used to treat heart failure, but wouldn't help relieve this patient's symptoms of severe ankle swelling.

30. D
Synchronised direct current (DC) cardioversion

This patient has presented with a supraventricular tachycardia, which started 2 hours ago. If any adverse signs such as: chest pain, hypotension (systolic blood pressure < 90 mmHg), heart failure, impaired consciousness or heart rate >200 bpm, are present then synchronised DC cardioversion should be used. Synchronised means that the shock is delivered at the same time that the R wave is produced on the electrocardiogram (ECG). If it is delivered during depolarisation of the myocardium it could cause ventricular fibrillation.

Desynchronised shocks are given where there is no cardiac output such as in ventricular fibrillation.

31. C
Sodium bicarbonate

This patient has taken a tricyclic antidepressant overdose. This is evident because of the antimuscarinic side effects she is experiencing: blurred vision, dry eyes, dry mouth and urinary retention (dull suprapubic mass). Others include dilated pupils, palpitations and constipation. Typical ECG changes are a broad complex tachycardia with a prolonged QTc. (QTc is the QT interval adjusted for the patient's heart rate.) It would also cause a metabolic acidosis with a raised anion gap. Treatment is to give intravenous sodium bicarbonate.

Haemodialysis would be used in overdoses of the following drugs: barbiturates, lithium, alcohol, salicylates and theophylline.

Calcium gluconate is given to stabilise the myocardium when ECG changes are caused by hyperkalaemia.

Intravenous insulin and dextrose is given to treat hyperkalaemia, and if it is refractory then haemodialysis may be used.

Digibind is a monoclonal antibody that binds to digoxin and is used in a digoxin overdose. Digoxin toxicity can present with nausea, vomiting, xanthopsia, confusion and arrhythmias.

Endocrine Questions

1. A known diabetic with poor glycaemic control presents with pain in his hips. On speaking to him the doctor manages to localise the pain to his quadriceps and around the pelvis. On examination there is marked wasting and weakness of the quadriceps. Which of the following drugs would be most likely to improve this patient's prognosis?

A. Prednisolone
B. Gabapentin
C. Baclofen
D. Cefuroxime
E. Intravenous immunoglobulins

2. A patient is brought into hospital by his friend. He appears confused and agitated. On examination he is sweating and tachycardic. Following an infusion of 50% dextrose he begins to feel better. Following this various investigations are carried out. As part of the investigations an insulin tolerance test is carried out. During this the C-peptide level is measured and remains the same throughout. What is the most likely underlying diagnosis?

A. Pituitary insufficiency
B. Addison's disease
C. Insulinoma
D. Metformin overdose
E. Insulin glargine overdose

3. A patient presents to hospital with confusion and whilst waiting to be seen she has a seizure. She is found to be hyponatraemic. She is deemed euvolaemic on examination. She recently attended her general practice (GP) surgery complaining of lethargy, weight gain, menorrhagia, dry skin and constipation. Considering the underlying diagnosis which of the following is most appropriate to treat her hyponatraemia?

A. Hydrocortisone
B. Tolvaptan
C. Levothyroxine
D. Insulin
E. Desmopressin

4. A patient presents to clinic with recent polydipsia, weight loss, constipation and non-specific bone pain. Whilst speaking to her it is noticed that she has a hoarse voice and it also becomes apparent that she has become very depressed recently. Her blood tests show the following:

Serum calcium:	3.1 mmol/L
Serum phosphate:	0.5 mmol/L
Serum parathyroid hormone (PTH):	0.2 pg/ml
Serum alkaline phosphatase (ALP):	300 U/L

Which of the following is likely to help confirm the underlying cause of this patient's hypercalcaemia?

A. Vitamin D levels
B. Urinary Bence-Jones proteins
C. Chest X-ray
D. Serum angiotensin converting enzyme (ACE)
E. Liver function tests

5. A 28-year-old woman presents to clinic with oligomenorrhea. On examination she is found to be overweight, have hirsutism and acne. Some investigations are requested and she is found to have normal thyroid stimulating hormone (TSH) and T4 levels. She reveals she is currently trying to conceive. Which of the following drugs would increase her chances of becoming pregnant?

A. Cyproterone acetate
B. Oestrogen
C. Spironolactone
D. Levothyroxine
E. Metformin

6. A young child presents to hospital following a seizure. A week prior to this he had seen his general practitioner (GP) due to a wheeze and muscle spasms. On examination he is of short stature with a round face and has short 4th and 5th metacarpals. Which of the following drugs should be used to treat the underlying cause of his symptoms?

A. Lanthanum
B. Hydrocortisone
C. Synthetic parathyroid hormone
D. Calcitriol
E. Cinacalcet

7. A patient presents with an asymptomatic lump in her neck. On examination it is found to be solitary lump, and there is also cervical lymphadenopathy. A radionucliotide scan shows that the nodule is cold, and blood tests show a raised level of thyroglobulin. What is the most likely underlying diagnosis?

A. Thyroid cyst
B. Thyroid adenoma
C. Papillary thyroid carcinoma
D. Follicular thyroid carcinoma
E. Medullary thyroid carcinoma

8. A woman develops Sheehan's syndrome post partum. Which of the following drugs should she be started on first?

A. Levothyroxine
B. Hydrocortisone
C. Fludrocortisone
D. Insulin
E. Growth hormone

9. A patient with a long-term history of brittle asthma presents to his general practitioner (GP) with increasing fatigue and dizzy spells. On examination his skin is of a normal pigment but he is found to have postural hypotension. When speaking to the GP it becomes apparent that recently he has not been very compliant with his oral prednisolone. The GP ordered some investigations, which of the following is most likely to be found?

A. Raised cortisol in response to a short synacthen test
B. 21-hydroxylase adrenal antibody positive
C. Undetectable adrenocorticotropic hormone (ACTH) levels
D. Raised fasting venous glucose
E. Normal renin: aldosterone ratio

10. A patient who was recently diagnosed with sleep apnoea and type 2 diabetes mellitus presents to his doctor with back pain, and pain in her left hand. On examination his skin appeared to be hyperpigmented and Tinel's test was positive. Which of the following investigations would confirm the underling diagnosis?

A. Short synathen test
B. Serum ferritin
C. Oral glucose tolerance test
D. Insulin tolerance test
E. Urinary beta human chorionic gonadotropin (HCG)

11. A 60-year-old male with a history of type 2 diabetes mellitus is diagnosed with hypertension following a 24-hour ambulatory monitoring of his blood pressure. He is prescribed a new drug to control his blood pressure. On review it is noticed that his glyacemic control has worsened. Which of the following drugs was he prescribed?

A. Amlodipine
B. Hydralazine
C. Bendroflumethiazide
D. Doxazosin
E. Ramipril

12. A young woman presents to her doctor with primary amenorrhea. When speaking the doctor notices she has a deep voice. On examination she appears to have increased musculature and appears dehydrated. Her routine blood tests show the following:

Serum sodium: 130 mmol/L
Serum potassium: 5.9 mmol/L
Serum urea: 9.0 mg/dL
Serum creatinine: 130 µmol/L

What is the most likely underlying diagnosis?

A. Hypothyroidism
B. Polycystic kidney disease
C. Prolactinoma
D. 21-hydroxylase deficiency
E. Conn's syndrome

13. A patient with poorly controlled diabetes mellitus presents with a two month history vomiting and diarrhoea, along with abdominal pain and bloating, which is worse after eating. He also notices that on standing from a seated position he often feels dizzy, and has fainted on two occasions. He is subsequently diagnosed with an autonomic neuropathy. Which of the following combinations of drugs would be most effective in treating this patient's symptoms?

A. Phenylephrine and domperidone
B. Dexamethasone and tetracycline
C. Fludrocortisone and erythromycin
D. Fludrocortisone and ciprofloxacin
E. Fludrocortisone and hyoscine butylbromide

14. A 75-year-old male who is currently being treated for schizophrenia presents to clinic with gynecomastia, galactorrhea and erectile dysfunction. On examination he is found to have a bitemporal hemianopia. Which of the following treatment regimes should be used to treat this patient's symptoms?

A. Stop his risperidone
B. Trans-sphenoidal surgery
C. Start cabergoline
D. Start ropinirol
E. Start tamoxifen

15. A 26-year-old female presents to her doctor with weight gain and oligomenorrhea. She is referred to an endocrinologist and treated for hypothyroidism with thyroxine. Her symptoms completely resolved and she lost the weight she had recently gained. During her follow-up the endocrinologist decides to screen for a few other causes of her initial symptoms and finds a raised level of prolactin, despite the patient being asymptomatic. Which of the following statements would explain these findings?

A. Her dose of thyroxine is too low
B. Her hypothyroidism was caused by pituitary stalk damage
C. She is currently taking metoclopramide
D. She has macroprolactin
E. She has underlying multiple endocrine neoplasia type 1

16. A patient presents to his doctor following a period of polydispia and polyuria. His blood tests show he is hypernatraemic. Once he is stabilised some investigations are carried out. These began with a water deprivation test. The results are as follows:

Urine osmolarity at the start:	180 mOsm/kg
Urine osmolarity after four hours:	210 mOsm/kg (normal >600 mOsm/kg)
Urine osmolarity after intranasal desmporessin:	220 mOsm/kg (normal >600 mOsm/kg)

Which of the following diagnoses may explain this patient's symptoms?

A. Addison's disease
B. Type 1 diabetes mellitus
C. Mutation of the V_2 receptor
D. Pituitary stalk damage
E. Conn's syndrome

17. A patient presents to an endocrinologist with recent weight gain and depression. On examination she is found to have central obesity with abdominal purple striae and proximal muscle weakness. A few investigations are requested:

48 hour dexamethasone suppression test:	Cortisol remained high
Adrenocorticotrophin (ACTH) level:	Raised
Corticotrophin releasing hormone (CRH) stimulation test:	Cortisol levels were unaffected

Considering the underlying diagnosis, which of the following investigations would be most useful?

A. Testing visual fields
B. Adrenal vein sampling
C. Bilateral inferior petrosal sinus blood sampling
D. Computed tomography (CT) scan of the chest, abdomen and pelvis
E. Oestrogen, progesterone, luteinising hormone (LH), follicle stimulating hormone (FSH) and testosterone levels

18. A 35-year-old male is diagnosed with gynecomastia. Which of the following drugs could be used to treat him?

A. Tamoxifen
B. Goserelin
C. Cyproterone acetate
D. Finasteride
E. Cimetidine

19. A 44-year-old woman presents to clinic with agitation, anxiety, sleep disturbance and recent weight loss. She also complains of always feeling hot. Which of the following is least consistent with the underling diagnosis?

A. Dry gritty eyes
B. Dry hair
C. Onycholysis
D. Irregularly irregular pulse
E. Hyporeflexia

20. A 30-year-old female with presents to clinic. The following blood tests were requested:

Serum sodium:	138 mmol/L
Serum potassium:	4.6 mmol/L
Serum urea:	5.0 mg/dL
Serum creatinine:	77 µmol/L
Serum calcium:	2.1 mmol/L
Serum phosphate:	1.8 mmol/L
Parathyroid hormone (PTH):	85 pg/ml

What is the most likely cause of her blood test results?

A. Parathyroid gland adenoma
B. Parathyroid gland hyperplasia
C. Chronic kidney disease
D. Vitamin D deficiency
E. Osteoporosis

21. A 23-year-old presents with reduced consciousness. Her mother reported that for the past few days she had been passing urine far more frequently than normal and also complained of dysuria. A urine dip shows the following:

Blood: −
Protein: −
Glucose: +++
Ketones: ++
Leucocytes: ++
Nitrites: ++

Which of the following is the most appropriate first step in this patient's management?

A. First dose of trimethoprim
B. Fixed rate insulin infusion
C. 1 litre of 0.9% saline STAT
D. Low molecular weight heparin
E. Catheterisation

22. A 30-year-old female presents to hospital with lethargy, fatigue and a two week history of weight loss. As part of her work up the junior doctor performs an electrocardiogram (ECG) which is entirely normal, and some blood tests. The blood tests show the following:

Serum sodium: 127 mmol/L
Serum potassium: 6.3 mmol/L
Serum urea: 5.0 mg/dL
Serum creatinine: 80 µmol/L
Thyroid function tests: All within normal range

Which of the following is the next most important step in this patient's management?

A. Intravenous hydrocortisone
B. Urine dip
C. Fixed rate insulin infusion
D. Intravenous calcium gluconate
E. Oral fludrocortisone

23. A 30-year-old female is diagnosed with Grave's disease and started on propranolol and carbimazole. Two weeks later she attends a follow up appointment and on questioning reveals she has had a sore throat for the past three days. Which of the following tests should be organised?

A. Full blood count
B. Peripheral blood film
C. Thyroid function tests
D. Short synacthen test
E. Laryngoscopy

24. A type 2 diabetic has difficulty controlling her blood sugar levels and therefore is referred by her general practitioner (GP) to see an endocrinologist. She has a past medical history of hypercholestrol-aemia and ischaemic heart disease, which has resulted in heart fail-ure. The endocrinologist starts a new drug. Two weeks later the patient returns to her GP complaining of ankle swelling, dyspnea and orthopnea. Which of the following drugs was started?

A. Metformin
B. Gliclazide
C. Acarbose
D. Pioglitazone
E. Exenatide

25. An elderly type 2 diabetic is found with reduced consciousness in his flat. He is known to be poorly controlled and is currently just taking sitagliptin, but has poor compliance. On examination he is extremely dehydrated, with dry mucus membranes and a capillary refill time of 5 seconds. His serum blood glucose is 55 mmol/L. Which of the following is this patient most at risk of?

A. Pulmonary oedmea
B. Myocardial infarction
C. Venous thromboembolism
D. Hypoglycemia
E. hypercalcemia

26. A 55-year-old male presents with confusion and a Glasgow Coma Scale (GCS) score of 11. His capillary glucose is taken and is unrecordable. His urine dip shows the following:

Leucocytes: –
Nitrites: –
Blood: –
Proetin: –
Ketones: –
Glucose: +++

The doctors are still awaiting the results of his baseline blood tests. Which of the following treatment regimes should be started immediately?

A. 1 litre of Hartmann's STAT
B. 1 litre of 0.9% saline STAT
C. 1 litre of 0.9% saline STAT, followed a bolus of 10 units of insulin
D. 1 litre of 0.9% saline STAT, followed by fixed insulin infusion of 0.1 units per kg per hour
E. 1 litre of 0.9% saline STAT and an insulin sliding scale

27. An 80-year-old lady with mild dementia is admitted with new onset confusion. Her observations are as follows: respiratory rate = 20 breaths per minute, heart rate = 120 bpm, blood pressure = 75/40 mmHg, temperature = 36.5°C. Her initial blood tests show a normal full blood count and a hypernatraemia with a serum sodium of 155 mmol/L. Which of the following fluids should be started?

A. Gelofusine
B. 0.45% saline and 4% dextrose
C. 0.9% saline
D. 5% dextrose
E. Human albumin solution

28. A 35-year-old male with a history of inflammatory bowel disease is admitted to hospital. He is made 'nil by mouth' and is unable to take his current oral medications, which consist of 20 mg of prednisolone once a day. He is prescribed intravenous hydrocortisone. How much hydrocortisone should he be given each day to equal his normal corticosteroid intake?

A. 20 mg
B. 40 mg
C. 60 mg
D. 80 mg
E. 100 mg

29. A 45-year-old diabetic lady presents to her doctor with sudden painless loss of vision in her left eye. On examination of the affected eye her red reflex is absent. Which of the following is the most likely diagnosis?

A. Cataract
B. Diabetic retinopathy
C. Central retinal artery occlusion
D. Central retinal vein occlusion
E. Vitreous haemorrhage

30. A 56-year-old man attends a general practitioner (GP) appointment following a recent diagnosis of type 2 diabetes mellitus. His GP has already started him on metformin and is gradually increasing the dose. His test results show the following:

Blood pressure: 130/80 mmHg
Total cholesterol: 3.8 mmol/L
Urine dip: normal
Urinary albumin/creatinine ratio: 7.2 mg/mmol

Which of the following medications should also be started?

A. Amlodipine
B. Ramipril
C. Atorvastatin
D. Benzafibrate
E. Gliclazide

Endocrine Answers

1. E
Intravenous immunoglobulins

This patient has developed diabetic amyotrophy, which is painful wasting of the quadriceps and pelvifemoral muscles. It is diagnosed by electrophysiology, which shows lumbosacral radiculopathy, plexopathy or proximal cural neuropathy. Intravenous immunoglobulins can be used in treatment, and it is also important to maintain good glycaemic control.

Gabapentin and baclofen can be used as third line treatments for diabetic neuropathy. Gabapentin was first developed as an anti-epileptic drug, but is now used to treat neuropathic pain.

Baclofen activates the GABA-B receptor, which causes hyperpolarisation of neurones and reduces their activity. It is used as a muscle relaxant in patients with spasticity, such as patients with multiple sclerosis or cerebral palsy.

Duloxetine is a serotonin-norepinephrine reuptake inhibitor (SNRI) used as first line treatment in diabetic neuropathy, often followed by amitriptyline.

Prednisolone is an oral corticosteroid, and should be avoided in patients with diabetes mellitus if possible, because it increases insulin resistance and can worsen their glycaemic control.

Cefuroxime is a second generation cephalosporin antibiotic.

2. C
Insulinoma

This patient had hypoglycemia, caused by an insulinoma. Insulinomas are endocrine tumours that secrete insulin and thus cause hypoglycemia. They present with fasting hypoglycemia, and symptoms of hypoglycemia (such as sweating, anxiety, tremor and hunger) upon fasting or exercise, that are relieved upon eating. Monitoring C-peptide levels during an insulin tolerance test is used to diagnose insulinomas. C-peptide is a protein that is produced by the Beta cells in the Islets of Langerhans, during the production of endogenous insulin. It allows us to differentiate as to whether insulin in the body is endogenous, or exogenous (where no C-peptide would be produced). Normally levels would decrease due to negative feedback mechanisms once exogenous insulin is given, but in an insulinoma, levels remain high.

Insulinomas can occur as part of MEN1 (multiple endocrine neoplasia type 1), which occurs due to a mutation in the tumour suppressor gene MEN-1. It causes parathyroid hyperplasia, pituitary prolactinomas and pancreatic tumours (such as insulinomas and gastrinomas).

Pituitary insufficiency and Addison's disease both cause hypoglycemia due to reduced levels of cortisol. In pituitary insufficiency all the pituitary hormones are deplete including ACTH, which leads to reduced cortisol. Addison's disease is due to dysfunction of the adrenal gland. Both conditions would present with low insulin (therefore a low C-peptide) and raised ketones.

Metformin is a biguanide used to treat type 2 diabetes mellitus. It doesn't cause hypoglycemia. The main groups of drugs that cause hypoglycemia are sulphonylureas, synthetic insulin and alcohol.

This case is not due to insulin glargine overdose, because synthetic insulin causes reduced levels of C-peptide, due to the negative feedback effects on the Beta cells.

3. C
Levothyroxine

This patient has severe hypothyroidism. This classically presents with tiredness, weight gain, dry skin, dry hair, and hair loss in the outer third of the eyebrows, hoarse voice, constipation and menorrhagia. If severe it can also cause dementia, a transudative pleural effusion, ascites, ataxia due to cerebellar pathology and congestive cardiac failure due to a dilated cardiomyopathy. Blood tests would show low thyroxine, and if severe may show a macrocytic anaemia and hyponatraemia. The causes of euvolaemic hyponatraemia include syndrome of inappropriate antidiuretic hormone (ADH) secretion (SIADH), water overload, glucocorticoid insufficiency and severe hypothyroisism.

Tolvaptan is a vaptan, which acts as a vasopressor receptor antagonist. It can be used to treat SIADH, which would present with a high urine osmolality and low serum osmolality.

Desmopressin is used as a vasopressin receptor agonist, and used to treat diabetes insipidus, which normally presents with hypernatraemia.

Insulin would be used in patients who have diabetes type 1, or type 2, which cannot be controlled with oral medication.

Hydrocortisone is a corticosteroid given in Addison's disease to replace the normal production of cortisol that has been lost. In Addison's disease patients present with lethargy, weight loss, dehydration, polyuria and polydipsia. Their blood tests would show hyperkalaemia, hyponatraemia and hypoglycemia.

4. C
Chest X-ray

This patient has an underlying malignancy, which has resulted in symptomatic hypercalcaemia. Hypercalcaemia presents with polyuria, polydipsia, anorexia, nausea and vomiting, abdominal pain, renal colic, bone pain, confusion, depression and psychosis. Squamous cell lung cancers are able to produce parathyroid hormone related peptide. This creates a similar picture to primary hyperparathyroidism with raised calcium, low phosphate and raised alkaline phosphatase (ALP), but it cannot be detected on the parathyroid hormone (PTH) assay, so PTH appears to be low. The malignancy has damaged the recurrent laryngeal nerve leading to a hoarse voice, and it has also caused weight loss.

Multiple myeloma is a malignant clonal proliferation of betalymophocyte derived plasma cells. This causes many problems including hypercalcaemia as a result of lytic bone lesions (which also cause pain and pathological fractures), renal failure, pancytopenia (which can lead to infections and bleeding), hyperviscosity and amyloidosis. Myeloma can be tested for by looking for Bence-Jones proteins in the urine, which is formed from the immunoglobulin light chains. Myeloma would cause a normal or low ALP.

Vitamin D excess can cause hypercalcaemia. There are different types of vitamin D supplements. The most likely to cause hypercalcaemia would be alfacalcidol, because it is already active and doesn't require conversion by 1-alpha-hydroxyalse in the kidneys. This is mainly used in kidney failure. In vitamin D excess the ALP is normal or low. Vitamin D is present in the form of cholecalciferol in the skin, is converted to calcidiol in the liver and calcitriol in the kidneys. Liver function tests may be required in hypocalcaemia to look for evidence of cirrhosis, which would lead to vitamin D not being converted from cholecalciferol to calcidiol.

Serum ACE is raised in sarcoidosis, which is another cause of hypercalcaemia. This can be used to help form a diagnosis of sarcoid. However due to the hoarse voice, lung cancer has to be ruled out first and therefore a chest X-ray is most appropriate.

5. E
Metformin

This patient has polycystic ovary syndrome (PCOS). This presents with oligomenorrhea, acne, hirsutism, weight gain and insulin resistance. It is caused by secretion of androgens from the ovaries. Tests show raised levels of testosterone, raised luteinising hormone (LH): follicle stimulating hormone (FSH) ratio, and decreased sex-hormone binding globulin. Spironolactone and cyproterone acetate are used as anti-androgen drugs to treat PCOS, but they are also teratogenic. Oestrogen can also be used in the form of the combined oral contraceptive pill, but would act as contraception. Levothyroxine is not required, but thyroid function tests should always be ordered, because hypothyroidism can also cause oligomenorrhea and weight gain. Metformin is often used to reduce insulin resistance, and can also increase the chance of pregnancy. The other drug often used is clomiphene, which is a selective oestrogen antagonist that acts on the pituitary gland, and thus increases the release of FSH, causing ovulation.

6. D
Calcitriol

This patient has pseudohypoparathyroidism and has symptomatic hypocalcaemia, which presents with muscle spasms, seizures, increased smooth muscle tone (causing wheeze and dysphagia), perioral paraesthesiae and anxiety. This is a condition caused by mutation in the parathyroid hormone (PTH) receptors, and thus it leads to a lack of response to PTH. It presents with short 4th and 5th metacarpals, short stature, round face and a reduced intelligence quotient (IQ). Tests show low calcium, raised phosphate and raised PTH. It is treated with calcium supplements and calcitrol. Synthetic PTH wouldn't work, due to the mutation in the receptors, but it can be used as treatment for hypoparathyroidism.

Cinacalcet mimics calcium and therefore acts to reduce the production of PTH. It is used in hyperparathyroidism.

Lanthanum is a phosphate binder, which is given to treat chronic kidney disease (CKD). In CKD there is a lack of vitamin D activation by the kidneys resulting in hypocalcaemia and increased release of PTH. This leads to secondary hyperparathyroidism and causes hypocalcaemia and hyperphosphataemia.

7. C
Papillary thyroid carcinoma

The differentials for a solitary nodule include malignancy, adenoma, cyst and a discrete nodule in a multinodular goitre. If the radionucliotide scan shows the nodule is cold, and hypofunctioning it is more likely to be malignant. Papillary neoplasms are the most common type of thyroid malignancy. They classically metastasise via the lymph nodes causing cervical lymphadenopathy, and spread to the lungs. Thyroglobulin is a tumour marker for both papillary tumours and follicular tumours. Follicular tumours are less common and they metastasise via the blood to the lungs and bone. Medullary neoplasms are found in multiple endocrine neoplasia type 2 (MEN2) and produce calcitonin, which can be used as a tumour marker.

8. B
Hydrocortisone

Sheehan's syndrome is where hypovolaemic shock due to post partum haemorrhage causes ischaemic necrosis of the pituitary gland and panhypopituitarism. In any cause of panhypopituitarism it is important to replace the corticosteroids first. If the thyroxine is replaced first it can lead to a crisis. Growth hormone is less important and often not required in adults. Neither insulin nor fludrocortisone are required as their production is not dependent on the pituitary gland.

9. E
Normal renin: aldosterone ration

This patient is on long-term high dose corticosteroids to treat his brittle asthma, which he has recently stopped taking and as a result has developed iatrogenic secondary adrenal insufficiency. This is due to suppression of the pituitary adrenal axis via corticosteroids activating the negative feedback pathway. This results in low adrenocorticotrophin (ACTH) levels, which in turn causes atrophy of the adrenal glands. If the corticosteroids are removed abruptly the adrenals are unable to produce sufficient hydrocortisone to replace the synthetic corticosteroids. The sudden lack of cortisol would lead to a rise in ACTH levels but the adrenals would not be able to respond.

The short synathen test is likely to be positive, with the cortisol levels being unable to increase in response to synthetic ACTH.

21-hydroxylase adrenal antibodies are only found in autoimmune Addison's disease.

The fasting venous glucose is likely to be low due to reduced cortisol levels.

The renin: aldosterone ratio would not be affected, as the mineralocorticoid pathway is not under control of ACTH.

In autoimmune Addison's disease the renin: aldosterone ratio would be raised, because the adrenals would not be able to respond to the release of renin, due to destruction of the zona granulosa. The renin : aldosterone ratio is also used to differentiate between primary hyperaldosteronism (where it is reduced), and secondary hyperaldosteronism (where it is raised).

10. C
Oral glucose tolerance test

This patient has acromegaly, which is caused by a pituitary tumour secreting growth hormone. It can present with coarse facial features, gum hypertrophy, macroglossia, obstructive sleep apnoea, growth of hands and feet, arthralgia, back pain, congestive cardiac failure, hyperpigmentation of the skin, acanthosis nigricans, carpal tunnel sydnrome and insulin resistance. Sleep apnoea can occur due to obstruction of the airflow due to expansion of the laryngeal cartilage, laryngeal dyspnea (which is fixed cords that can also lead to dysphonia) and macroglossia. The oral glucose tolerance test is used to diagnose acromegaly. Normally when a bolus of glucose is given the levels of growth hormone would decrease, however in acromegaly they remain high.

The short synathen test can be used to test for Addison's disease.

Ferritin levels may be used as part of a diagnosis of hereditary haemochromatosis, which can present with diabetes, slate grey skin, arthralgia, and liver cirrhosis but is not associated with carpal tunnel syndrome.

Urinary HCG is the pregnancy test. Pregnancy can lead to gestational diabetes and cause carpal tunnel syndrome, but wouldn't cause the other symptoms described.

Insulin tolerance test can be used to diagnose many conditions including growth hormone deficiency. This often goes unnoticed in adults, but in children would cause reduced growth.

11. C
Bendroflumethiazide

This patient has been prescribed Bendroflumethiazide, which is a thiazide diuretic. One of the side effects of thiazide diuretics is that they can increase blood glucose levels. It is also thought that beta-blockers have a similar effect. The first choice antihypertensive in all diabetic patients is an ACE inhibitor (such as ramipril), because of its protective effect on the kidneys. Ramipril can worsen kidney function in patients who have renal artery stenosis, so creatinine levels must be monitored when the medication is first started.

Amlodipine is a dihydropyridine calcium channel blocker, and is the first line antihypertensive medication in Afro-Caribbean patients, and patients over 55 years old who are not diabetic. Its side effects include facial flushing, tachycardia, ankle swelling and headaches.

Doxazosin is an alpha-blocker and used as a third line antihypertensive drug. Its side effects include postural hypotension, and nasal stuffiness.

Hydralazine is a fourth line antihypertensive drug. Its precise mechanism is still unknown, but it acts by causing vasodilation. It is one of the medications that can cause drug induced lupus.

12. D
21-hydroxylase deficiency

This patient has congenital adrenal hyperplasia (CAH), which is caused by either a deficiency in 21-hydroxylase, or 11β-hydroxylase. These enzymes are present in the adrenals and are used to produce corticosteroids and mineralocorticoids. Without these enzymes there is a lack of cortisol and instead over-production of androgens. These cause virilism, muscular hypertrophy and cliteromegaly. The lack of cortisol for negative feedback leads to high levels of adrenocorticotrophin (ACTH), and adrenal hyperplasia. 21-hydroxylase deficiency is also known as salt wasting CAH due to the lack of production of mineralocorticoids. This causes dehydration and electrolyte imbalances (hyponatraemia and hyperkalaemia). 11β-hydroxylase deficiency is salt sparing as it leads to production of 11-deoxycorticosterone, which is a mineralocorticoid. In CAH 11-deoxycorticosterone is not under negative feedback like aldosterone, and is not controlled by the renin-angiotensin system. Instead it's levels are controlled by ACTH. It causes salt retention and hypertension.

Hypothyroidism can cause menorrhagia, whereas hyperthyroidism is more likely to cause amenorrhea.

Polycystic ovary syndrome (PCOS) can present with similar symptoms due to raised levels of androgens such as amenorrhea, acne, hirsutism, but it wouldn't have the electrolyte imbalances seen above.

A prolactinoma would cause hyperprolactinaemia and can lead to amenorrhea, galactorrhea, low libedo, vaginal dryness, and weight gain.

Conn's syndrome is also known as primary hyperaldosteronism, caused by increased aldosterone production from the adrenal glands. It causes hypertension, hypernatraemia and hypokalaemia.

13. C
Fludrocortisone and erythromycin

This patient has developed autonomic neuropathy due to poorly controlled diabetes. This has caused postural hypotension (which leads to dizziness and syncope on standing) and gastroparesis (which causes vomiting, early satiety and bloating after meals). Postural hypotension is treated with fludrocortisone. This is a mineralocorticoid, which acts to cause salt and water retention, thus maintaining a stable blood pressure.

Gastroparesis is treated by use of pro-kinetic drugs such as domperidone (an antiemetic) and erythromycin (a macrolide antibiotic). Therefore out of the combinations listed fludrocortisone and erythromycin is the only combination that would treat these underlying conditions.

Tetracycline could be used if it was thought this patient had bacterial overgrowth as a result of gastroparesis. Bacterial overgrowth would present with diarrhoea, steatorrhea and malabsorption.

Phenylephrine is an alpha 1-adrenoceptor agonist, used as a decongestant. This is not used to treat postural hypotension, however midodrine (which has the same mechanism) can be used.

Hyoscine butylbromide is an antimuscarinic drug, which can be used as an antiemetic (especially to treat motion sickness) and can be used to treat stomach cramps.

Dexamethasone (a potent corticosteroid) also has antiemetic properties, and is especially effective in patients with nausea and vomiting as a result of chemotherapy treatments.

14. B
Trans-sphenoidal surgery

This patient has a macroprolactinoma. This is evident in his symptoms of hyperprolactinaemia such as gynecomastia, galactorrhea and erectile dysfunction; and the bitemporal hemianopia. This has been caused by compression of the optic chiasm and can occur in any pituitary tumour (which affects the superior visual fields) or a craniopharyngioma (which affects the inferior visual fields). Due to the visual disturbance, surgery is the most appropriate option.

Cabergoline is a dopamine receptor agonist used to reduce prolactin secreation. This can be used in patients with microprolactinomas, however it is contraindicated in patients with schizophrenia, because the majority of antipsychotic treatments involving dopamine receptor antagonists.

Ropinirole is also a dopamine receptor agonist, but is used to treat Parkinson's disease.

Risperidone is an atypical antipsychotic, and one of its side effects is hyperprolactinaemia. It acts by the antagonism of dopamine D2-receptors. Dopamine acts on the anterior pituitary gland to inhibit secretion of prolactin. Therefore if the receptors are blocked, more is released causing hyperprolactinaemia. However it is not the underlying cause in this case because of the presence of a bitemporal hemianopia.

Tamoxifen is a selective oestrogen receptor antagonist, used to treat gynecomastia, and breast cancer which is positive for oestrogen receptors on histology. It doesn't act on receptors in the bone and therefore doesn't cause osteoporosis.

15. D
She has macroprolactin

Macroprolactin is a physiologically inactive protein that is bound to IgG. It is removed slowly by the kidneys due to its size and causes a falsely elevated prolactin result. The assay used cannot tell the difference between macroprolactin and prolactin. Despite the elevated levels the patient wouldn't experience any symptoms because the macroprolactin is inactive. The test requested by the doctor was an asymptomatic screen; therefore this is most likely to be the cause.

All the other causes listed are causes of hyperprolactinaemia, but would all cause symptoms such as galactorrhea, oligomenorrhea, low libido, vaginal dryness and weight gain. If she had pituitary stalk damage she would also experience other symptoms of panhypopituitarism, such as those associated with Addison's disease, which include polyuria, polydipsia, nausea, vomiting, fatigue and abdominal pain.

Multiple endocrine neoplasia type 1 causes a prolactinoma, pancreatic tumour and parathyroid hyperplasia and therefore would also present with symptoms of hypercalcaemia, and symptoms related to a pancreatic tumour, such as peptic ulcers if a gastrinoma was present.

If her thyroxine level were too low, she would still have symptoms of hypothyroidism. She is currently asymptomatic, so this is not the case.

Metoclopramide can cause hyperprolactinaemia, because it is a dopamine D2-receptor antagonist and therefore blocks the inhibitory dopamine affects on the anterior pituitary gland. However this would cause symptoms of raised prolactin.

16. C
Mutation of the V_2 receptor

This patient has nephrogenic diabetes insipidus. This is where the kidneys don't respond to vasopressin. This presents with polydipsia, polyuria and hypernatraemia. It can be distinguished from cranial diabetes insipidus because it doesn't respond to desmopressin during the water deprivation test.

Therefore during the water deprivation test the urine remains a low osmolality despite dehydration and use of desmopressin. The causes of nephrogenic diabetes insipidus are: congenital mutation in the V_2 receptor found in the kidneys (V_1 is found on the blood vessels), hypercalcaemia, hypokalaemia, chronic kidney disease and lithium.

Pituitary stalk damage is a cause of cranial diabetes insipidus. Vasopressin is produced in the hypothalamus and moves down neurones to the posterior pituitary gland where it is realised. Damage to the stalk prevents this from occurring. Other causes include damage to the hypothalamus (such as in trauma, ischaemic or haemorrhagic stroke, and cranial tumours) and also damage to the pituitary gland via similar mechanisms.

Diabetes mellitus would also present with polyuria and polydipsia but is more likely to cause hyponatraemia due to osmolar diuresis. Also the body attempts to maintain serum osmolality (serum osmolality = 2[sodium + potassium] + glucose + urea), and therefore will selectively excrete sodium if the levels of glucose begin to rise. So in diabetes mellitus the body counteracts the affect of a rising glucose by losing sodium. Therefore patients presenting in diabetic ketoacidosis often present with hyponatraemia.

Conn's syndrome is where there is an adrenal adenoma that secretes excessive aldosterone. This causes salt and fluid retention. Patients present with hypertension, that is difficult to control, hypernatraemia, hypokalaemia and a metabolic alkalosis. They don't present with polyuria, polydipsia and dehydration.

Addison's disease is caused by autoimmune destruction of the adrenal glands, and would present with a low sodium, high potassium and low glucose. This occurs due to a lack of cortisol production.

17. D
Computed tomography (CT) scan of the chest, abdomen and pelvis

This patient has developed Cushing's disease as a result of ectopic adrenocorticotrophin (ACTH) production. Cushing's disease presents with weight gain, central obesity, purple straie, buffalo hump, proximal muscle weakness, rounded facial appearance, acne and hirsutism. It can cause hypertension, peptic ulcers, osteoporosis, insulin resistance, pancreatitis, cataracts, glaucoma and bone marrow suppression.

This patient has raised ACTH levels. In Cushing's syndrome (due to an adrenal adenoma, or adrenal hyperplasia), ACTH would be undetectable due to a negative feedback mechanism. Therefore this is Cushing's disease, and the ACTH is either being produced by the pituitary gland or by ectopic production. If the production of ACTH were from the pituitary gland it would be suppressed by high doses of dexamethasone, due to negative feedback. Ectopic production doesn't respond to high dose dexamethasone. Also ectopic production of ACTH will not respond to synthetic corticotrophin-realeasing hormone (CRH), therefore the levels of cortisol would not increase. If production were from the pituitary gland then it would respond to a CRH stimulation test.

Causes of ectopic production include a paraneoplastic syndrome due to small cell lung cancer, and therefore a CT Chest, abdomen and pelvis is most useful to look for the underlying cancer.

Testing visual fields would be important if there was pituitary production, as this would cause a bitemporal hemianopia.

Both the CRH stimulation test and bilateral inferior petrosal sinus blood sampling can be used to confirm pituitary overproduction of ACTH. CRH stimulation test is where synthetic CRH is given and then patients are tested for a rise in cortisol. Ectopic production doesn't respond to CRH. Bilateral inferior petrosal sinus blood sampling takes blood directly from the veins draining from the pituitary gland and looks for a rise in ACTH in that blood, which would indicate the presence of an ACTH producing pituitary adenoma.

Adrenal vein sampling can be used to distinguish between a solitary adrenal adenoma and bilateral adrenal hyperplasia. It looks at the level of cortisol being produced in each adrenal gland. More commonly imaging such as a CT or magnetic resonance imaging (MRI) scan of the adrenals is used to make the distinction.

Oestrogen, progesterone, LH, FSH and testosterone levels would be requested if a diagnosis of polycystic ovary syndrome (PCOS) were suspected. This can also present with weight gain, but would also present with other features such as oligomenorrhea and wouldn't cause purple striae.

18. A
Tamoxifen

Tamoxifen is a selective oestrogen receptor antagonist. It can be used to treat gynecomastia and breast cancer. Its side effects include fatty liver disease and increased risk of venous thromboembolism.

All the other drugs listed cause gynecomastia. Goserelin is a gonadotrophin-releasing hormone (GnRH) receptor agonist, and cyproterone acetate is an androgen receptor antagonist both of which can be used to treat prostate cancer. Finasteride is a 5α-reductase inhibitor, used in benign prostatic hyperplasia, and cimetidine is an H_2-receptor antagonist used to reduce production of stomach acid. Other drug causes of gynaecomastia include digoxin, spironolactone and the overuse of levothyroxine.

19. E
Hyporeflexia

This patient has hyperthyroidism. Grave's disease is the most common cause of hyperthyroidism and is the most likely cause of hyperthyroidism in this case because this patient is a young woman. Grave's disease occurs due to the production of autoantibodies that activate the thyroid stimulating hormone (TSH) receptors.

The only finding listed, which is not consistent with Grave's disease, is hyporeflexia. In hypothyroidism there may be a slowed relaxation phase of reflexes. The dry gritty eyes are as a result of lid retraction and exophthalmos. This occurs due to thyroid eye disease, as a result of antigens in the extra-orbital muscles being similar to the TSH receptors. Therefore the autoantibodies cause retro-orbital inflammation.

Dry hair and onycholysis can be found in both hyper and hypothyroidism. The irregularly irregular pulse is due to atrial fibrillation can occur in hyperthyroidism.

20. D
Vitamin D deficiency

This patient has developed secondary hyperparathyroidism. This is where there is appropriate over activity of the parathyroid glands as a result of hypocalcaemia. Blood tests show hypocalcaemia, hyperphoshataemia and raised PTH. This can be caused by either vitamin D deficiency or chronic kidney disease. The reason it is more likely to be vitamin D deficiency is because this patient's kidney function appears to be normal.

Tertiary hyperparathryroidism occurs following prolonged secondary hyperparathyroidism as a result of chronic kidney disease. The parathyroid glands act autonomously, and independent of negative feedback. This results in hypercalcaemia and a raised PTH.

Both parathyroid gland adenoma and hyperplasia cause primary hyperparathyroidism. This presents with raised calcium, raised PTH and a low phosphate.

Osteoporosis doesn't create any electrolyte imbalances and this would be rare in a patient this young as she is very unlikely to have gone through the menopause.

21. C
1 litre of 0.9% saline STAT

This patient has developed diabetic ketoacidosis (DKA). This is defined as the presence of a metabolic acidosis with raised ketones and hyperglycemia. This occurs due to a lack of insulin production in type 1 diabetic patients. The lack of insulin leads to a reduction in cellular glucose uptake and therefore the liver converts fatty acids to ketones by gluconeogenisis. DKA can be precipitated by a number of causes, the most common being infection. This patient's DKA is most likely to have been precipitated by a urinary tract infection, hence the presence of leucocytes and nitrites in the urine. Other precipitants include non-compliance with medications, other drugs (such as alcohol, cocaine, steroids, antipsychotics), pancreatitis and pregnancy.

Despite this patient having a urinary tract infection the priority is to treat the DKA. These patients become severely dehydrated due to osmotic diuresis. The priority is fluid replacement. Therefore 1 litre 0.9% saline STAT, should be given. Followed by a fixed rate insulin infusion of 0.1 units/kg/hour, along with meticulous monitoring of serum glucose, pH, bicarbonate and potassium.

Low molecular weight heparin should also be given, as this patient is likely to be dehydrated and therefore at risk of developing a venous thromboembolism.

Catheterisation is likely to be required to monitor urine output and fluid balance.

Trimethoprim is an antibiotic often used to treat urinary tract infections. She is likely to be started on an antibiotic but fluid resuscitation is still the priority.

22. A
Intravenous hydrocortisone

This patient has Addison's disease, which is where there is insufficient production of hydrocortisone in the adrenals. It presents with polyuria, polydipsia, abdominal pain, nausea and vomiting, weight loss, lethargy and fatigue. Blood tests classically show hyponatraemia, hyperkalaemia, and hypoglycemia. There may also be a metabolic acidosis with a normal anion gap. The electrolyte imbalances occur as a result of a lack of mineralocorticoids and hypoglycemia due to a lack of corticosteroids. In this case the treatment of choice is intravenous hydrocortisone. Oral fludrocortisone is used to replace the mineralocorticoids and would be initiated only once the patient has been stabalised with hydrocortisone and intravenous fluids.

This patient also has hyperkalaemia. This can lead to fatal cardiac arrhythmias. It starts off by causing tall, tented T waves, followed by small P waves and a broadened QRS complex, which eventually becomes sinusoidal and patients can develop ventricular fibrillation. Calcium gluconate should be given if ECG changes are present, as it can stabilise the myocardium and prevent ventricular arrhythmias. However this patient doesn't have ECG changes consistent with hyperkalaemia. If calcium gluconate were to be given in this setting it could destabilise the myocardium.

A urine dip would be more useful if this patient was suspected to have diabetes and developed a diabetic ketoacidosis, which can also present with weight loss and lethargy.

> Intravenous insulin can be given to treat hyperkalaemia, as it causes the cells to increase their uptake of serum potassium. However it must be given with 50% dextrose, to prevent hypoglyce-mia, which could be fatal. Other drugs that can be used include nebulised salbutamol, which also increases cellular uptake of potassium, and calcium resonium, which binds to potassium in the gut and reduces its absorption.

23. A
Full blood count

This patient has recently been started on carbimazole, which acts on the thyroid to reduce production of thyroxine. One of its side effects is agran-ulocytosis. This patient has presented with a sore throat, which could be a sign of infection, therefore it is important to check this patient's neutrophil levels with a full blood count. Other drug causes of agranulocytosis include propylthiouracil and clozapine.

A peripheral blood film can be used in haematological conditions such as acute myeloid leukaemia, which may show evidence of blast cells, however in this case it is not helpful.

Thyroid function tests would be used to monitor the patient's response to thyroxine, but this isn't the priority in this patient.

Short synacthen test is used to diagnose Addison's disease.

Laryngoscopy would be a detailed way of looking at the throat and vocal cords if any pathology was suspected. If this patient had a chronic sore throat this may be required, but for now the priority is to rule out agranulocytosis.

24. D
Pioglitazone

Pioglitazone is a thiazolindinedione drug that acts by activation of PPARgamma. Its side effects include fluid retention, osteoporosis, deranged liver function tests and an increased risk of bladder cancer. Due to these side effects its use is contraindicated in osteoporosis and congestive cardiac failure. Its side effect of fluid retention can be potentiated by co-prescription of insulin. This patient has developed worsening heart failure and is likely to have been prescribed pioglitazone.

Metformin is a biguanide and its side effects include abdominal pain, diarrhoea, and rarely lactic acidosis and vitamin B12 deficiency.

Gliclazide (which is a sulphonylurea) and subcutaneous insulin can both cause hypoglycemia and weight gain.

Exenatide is a glucagon like peptide 1 (GLP-1) analogue, which is given via a subcutaneous injection and acts by augmenting the actions of insulin. It slows the rate of digestion, thus increasing satiety and can help aid weight loss.

Acarbose is an alpha-glucosidase inhibitor, which prevents the breakdown of starch. Its side effects include bloating, stomach cramps and diarrhoea. Due to this, patients are often not very compliant with taking this medication.

25. C
Venous thromboembolism

This patient has developed a hyperglycemic hyperosmolar non-ketotic coma (HONK), which has more recently been renamed as a hyperosmolar hyperglycemic state (HHS). This occurs in poorly controlled type 2 diabetics. It leads to a gradual build up of serum glucose, often over the course of a week or longer. It presents with reduced consciousness, severe dehydration, and high glucose levels (typically much higher than those seen in diabetic ketoacidosis). Due to severe dehydration these patients are at risk of venous thromboembolism and therefore they should receive low molecular weight heparin as part of their treatment. They require gradual fluid resuscitation to avoid rapid changes in electrolytes and fluid shifts. These patients are severely dehydrated and therefore they are unlikely to become fluid overloaded and develop pulmonary oedema. Intravenous insulin can be started once the serum glucose no longer reduces with just fluid resuscitation.

These patients do not usually develop ketoacidosis, because there is still endogenous insulin present and therefore gluconeogenesis and production of ketones doesn't occur.

Hypoglycemia could occur once insulin is started, but not before. Sitagliptin is a dipeptidyl peptidase 4 (DPP-4) inhibitor and prevents the breakdown of glucagon like peptide 1 (GLP-1). Unlike sulphonylureas it doesn't cause weight gain or hypoglycemia.

26. B
1 litre of 0.9% saline

This patient has developed a hyperglycemic hyperosmolar non-ketotic coma (HONK), which has more recently been renamed as a hyperosmolar hyperglycemic state (HHS). This occurs in poorly controlled type 2 diabetics. It leads to a gradual build up of serum glucose, and due to the presence of insulin there is no ketone production. This gives the results of high levels of glucose and no ketones in the urine. These patients require slow fluid resuscitation with 0.9% saline. Insulin shouldn't be started until the patient's serum potassium is known. Giving insulin could precipitate hypokalaemia and cause life-threatening arrhythmias. When insulin is started, it would be started as a sliding scale rather than a fixed infusion, which is given, in diabetic ketoacidosis (DKA). 0.9% saline is preferred over Hartmann's in both HONK and DKA, because Hartmann's contains lactate and can worsen the metabolic acidosis.

27. C
0.9% saline

This patient is hypotensive and therefore requires fluid resuscitation. She is also hypernatremic, and therefore rescuitation with 0.9% saline is preferred. This is hypotonic in this patient and would cause less marked fluid shifts. Once the patient's blood pressure normalises the hyponatraemia must be corrected. If patients can take fluids orally then this should be encouraged, otherwise the fluid of choice is a slow infusion of 5% dextrose. Plasma sodium levels and urine output can guide the rate that intravenous fluids are given.

Human albumin solution acts as a colloid. It is most commonly used in patients who have liver cirrhosis and ascites, in an attempt to restore their serum albumin levels.

Gelofusine is a colloid plasma expander which is not commonly used because of the risk of anaphylatic reactions.

0.45% saline and 4% dextrose can be used in daily fluid maintenance and is sometimes preferred as it contains less sodium than 0.9% saline.

28. D
80 mg

Patients who are unable to take their oral corticosteroids must be converted to intravenous corticosteroids to prevent an Addisonian crisis. Hydrocortisone can be converted to prednsiolone by dividing the dose by four. Therefore 20mg of prednsiolone is equal to 80 mg of hydrocortisone. Other conversions are written below:

Hydrocortisone = Prednsiolone/4
Hydrocortisone = Methylprednisolone/5
Hydrocortisone = Dexamethasone/26.6

29. E
Vitreous haemorrhage

This presents with sudden painless loss of vision, and is caused by the rupture of a vessel in the retina. One of the risk factors for this is new vessel formation, which can occur in diabetes mellitus. Other causes include retinal tears, retinal detachment and trauma. If retinal detachment is the underlying cause, flashes and floaters may precede the loss of vision. If the bleed were large enough to obscure vision, it would also lead to an absent red reflex.

Other causes of a sudden painless loss of vision include: central retinal artery occlusion, central retinal vein occlusion and retinal detachment. Central retinal artery occlusion would still have a normal red reflex and ophthalmoscopy would show a pale retina with a cherry red spot at the macula. Central retinal vein occlusion would also have a normal red reflex, and ophthalmoscopy would show a stormy sunset appearance.

Diabetic retinopathy is another complication of diabetes and it would present with a gradual painless loss of vision that would occur over many years.

Cataract formation is also a complication of diabetes and would present with gradual painless loss of vision. Classically it would cause blurred vision, loss of depth perception (stereopsis) and a dazzle/glare when looking into bright lights at night.

30. B
Ramipril

It is important that diabetic patients are regularly followed up and their risk factors for vascular disease are modified. These include smoking cessation, blood pressure control, control of serum cholesterol, good glycaemic control and monitoring renal function. In this patient the most alarming test result is a raised urinary albumin/creatinine ratio. Any value above three requires intervention with either an angiotensin converting enzyme (ACE) inhibitor or an angiotensin II receptor blocker. These drugs should be prescribed even if the blood pressure is normal as they protect the kidneys. Blood pressure management in diabetes should always start with prescription of an ACE inhibitor before any other drug for this reason.

In diabetic patients the aim is for their total serum cholesterol to be less than 4 mmol/L and low density lipoprotein (LDL) cholesterol to be less than 2 mmol/L. If this is not the case then they should be started on a statin. Fibrates such as benzafibrate can be used to reduce serum triglycerides and increased high density lipoprotein (HDL) cholesterol levels.

This patient may require a sulphonylurea such as gliclazide in the future. However, he has just been started on metformin, and it would be wise to see how his glycaemic control is on his current medication, before adding in new medications.

Gastrointestinal Questions

1. A patient being treated for Crohn's disease is about to be started on infliximab. He is currently suffering from bloody diarrhoea and multiple fistulae. He doesn't report any chest pain or a cough. Which single set of investigations should be carried out before this patient begins this new medication?

A. Mantoux test and chest X-ray
B. Interferon gamma release assay and chest X-ray
C. Sputum cultures stained with a Ziehl-Neelsen stain
D. Liver function tests and urea and electrolytes
E. Nerve conduction studies

2. A 30-year-old man with a history ulcerative colitis was being treated with mesalazine, but recently had to be started on a short course of steroids and azathioprine in an attempt to control his symptoms. He is brought into hospital by his son following a three-day history of severe epigastric pain. He has also vomited twice and been producing fowl smelling stool that is difficult to flush. He is peripherally shut down and his blood results are as follows.

Haemoglobin:	136 g/L
White cell count:	15×10^9/L
Serum sodium:	135 mmol/L
Serum potassium:	4.5 mmol/L
Serum bilirubin:	11 µmol/l
Serum alanine aminotransferase (ALT):	152 U/L
Serum alkaline phosphatase (ALP):	94 IU/L
Serum amylase:	676 U/L

What is the underlying diagnosis?

A. Acute pancreatitis
B. Leaking abdominal aortic aneurysm
C. Addison's disease
D. Perforated duodenal ulcer
E. Inferior myocardial infarction

3. A 40 year old gentleman presents to his doctor with a rash on his left leg. The rash is red and hot to touch. He is diagnosed with cellulitis and given a course of antibiotics. Three weeks after completing the antibiotics he presents to his doctor with yellow sclera, puritis, dark urine and pale stools. Which of the following antibiotics was he prescribed?

A. Clindamycin
B. Phenoxymethylpenicillin
C. Trimethoprim
D. Flucloxacillin
E. Erythromycin

4. A 30-year-old woman with a history of pernicious anaemia is being investigated for unexplained raised transaminases (serum aspartate aminotransferase [AST] and alanine aminotransferase [ALT]). She later develops a fever, malaise, puritis and amenorrhoea. A liver screen is requested. Which of the following is most likely to be found?

A. Viral hepatitis
B. Positive anti-smooth muscle antibody
C. Raised IgM
D. Raised alpha-fetoprotein
E. Raised ferritin

5. A 72-year-old woman with a background of alcoholic liver cirrhosis is being treated for puritis with a new medication. She returns to clinic for review complaining of a non-specific bone pain that is spread all over her body. As she leaves the doctor notices she has a waddling gait. A bone profile shows hypocalcaemia, hypophosphataemia, a raised alkaline phosphatase and a low vitamin D level. Which of the following drugs was she prescribed?

A. Naltrexone
B. Codeine phosphate
C. Colestyramine
D. Ursodeoxycholic acid
E. Acamprosate

6. A 40-year-old male presents to his general practitioner (GP) with generalised fatigue, polydipsia and polyuria. He also states that he has been getting pain in his joints recently. On examination the patient's skin appears to be pigmented. His only significant family history is that his grandfather passed away at the age of 43 as a result of liver disease. His initial blood tests show deranged liver function. Which of the following investigations would be most sensitive and specific with regard to confirming the underlying diagnosis?

A. Short synacthen test
B. Fasting venous glucose
C. Liver biopsy with periodic acid–Schiff (PAS) stain
D. Liver biopsy with pearl stain
E. Serum ferritin

7. An intravenous drug user was recently treated for cellulitis using oral clindamycin. During his treatment he developed a fever, severe abdominal pain, and diarrhoea with blood and mucus present. Unfortunately he later developed peritonitis and died as a result of colonic perforation. Which of the following is most likely to be found at post-mortem during examination of the colon?

A. Pseudomembranous colitis
B. Cobble stoning
C. Pseudopolyposis
D. Colonic fibrosis
E. Serosal fat wrapping

8. A 40-year-old woman with a previous history of Grave's disease presents to her general practitioner (GP) with jaundice and puritis. She also describes recently having dark coloured urine and pale stools. On examination she is found to have ascites, xanthelasma and xanthemata. Her initial blood tests show deranged liver function and a raised IgM. Considering the underlying diagnosis, what is most likely to be found in a biopsy of the liver?

A. Fibrous obliterative cholangitis
B. Granulomas around the bile ducts
C. Ground glass hepatocytes
D. Steatohepatitis
E. Interface hepatitis

9. A patient presents to hospital with intermittent crushing chest pain, which is associated with dysphagia. The pain is relieved 20 minutes after using a glycerl trinitrate (GTN) spray. A barium swallow is conducted. Which of the following is likely to be found?

A. Bird beak appearance
B. Dilated tapering oesophagus
C. Cork screw oesophagus
D. Hiatus hernia
E. Zenker's diverticulum

10. A patient known to have angina pectoris was recently prescribed a new medication. He presents with severe dysphagia and retrosternal chest pain. After ruling out a cardiac cause for his pain he undergoes an endoscopy which shows severe oesophageal and gastric ulceration. Which of the following medications was recently started?

A. Atorvastatin
B. Bisoprolol
C. Clopidogrel
D. Diltiazem
E. Nicorandil

11. A patient recently had a gallstone removed by use of endoscopic retrograde cholangio-pancreatography (ECRP). Following the procedure the patient remained in hospital to recover. During this period he developed severe epigastric pain, which radiated to his back. This was followed by vomiting and on examination he was found to be tachycardic and hypotensive. Which of the following is the correct initial management for this patient?

A. Cefuroxime and metronidazole
B. Insertion of a nasogastric tube and intravenous 0.9% saline
C. Domperidone and diclofenac
D. Cholecystectomy
E. Emergency laparotomy

12. A 25-year-old female presents to clinic with an 8-month history of watery diarrhoea. She is also currently being investigated for amenorrhea by a gynaecologist. On examination she appears underweight, and her abdomen is soft and non-tender. A colonoscopy is scheduled. The macroscopic appearance of the colon was normal, but a biopsy showed brown pigmentation in the macrophages in the lamina propria (also known as lipofuscin-laden macrophages). What is the most likely underlying diagnosis?

A. Lymphocytic colitis
B. Melanosis coli
C. Whipple's disease
D. Entamoeba histolytica
E. Irritable bowel syndrome

13. A patient presents to clinic with weight loss and jaundice. Urinalysis showed raised urinary bilirubin, but absent urobilinogen. Which of the following is most likely to be causing this patient's jaundice?

A. Gilbert's syndrome
B. Budd-Chiari syndrome
C. Hepatocellular carcinoma
D. Cholangiocarcinoma
E. Simvastatin use

14. A patient presents to his doctor with a 6-month history of diarrhoea. He states there is no blood or mucus present in his stool, but it is difficult to flush and has an offensive smell. He also reported abdominal pain, bloating and weight loss. His initial blood tests show a normocytic anaemia. Which of the following blood tests would be most sensitive at diagnosing the underlying condition?

A. Anti-endomysial antibody
B. Anti-tissue transglutaminase antibody
C. Anti-gliadin antibody
D. Perinuclear anti-neutrophil cytoplasmic antibodies (P-ANCA)
E. Anti-saccharomyces cerevisiae antibody (ASCA)

15. A 23-year-old female who recently started a course of fluoxetine for depression presents to the emergency department with severe generalised abdominal pain. On examination the patient is pyrexial, tachycardic and hypertensive. She has complete weakness and loss of sensation in both upper limbs. Her routine bloods show she is hyponatraemic. Initial investigations show her urinary prophobilinogens are raised. Which of the following drugs should be used to reduce this patient's blood pressure?

A. Indapamide
B. Hydralazine
C. Methyldopa
D. Verapamil
E. Labetalol

16. A patient presents to clinic with an extremely itchy blistering rash on her elbows. She also has a previous 6-month history of weight loss and diarrhoea. A jejunal biopsy was taken as part of the investigations and showed flattening of the villi and crypt elongation. Considering the underlying diagnosis, which of the following treatment regimes should be used to treat this patient's rash?

A. Prednisolone
B. Ciclosporin
C. Azathioprine
D. Dapsone
E. Topical hydrocortisone

17. A 43-year-old woman presents to hospital with acute severe abdominal pain and vomiting. On examination she is found to have ascites and tender hepatomegaly. She has a previous history of multiple deep vein thromboses. Which of the following options is most appropriate in this patient's management?

A. Toxicology screen
B. Start N-acetylcysteine
C. Ultrasound scan of the abdomen
D. Intravenous cefuroxime and metronidazole
E. Arrange transfer to local center for a liver transplant

18. A 20-year-old male presents to his doctor with a 2-year history of blood in his stool. He says it has been intermittent and he hasn't experienced any other changes in his bowel habits. On systems review it became apparent that he has had recurrent nose bleeds since a young age. The doctor carries out a full examination of the patient. On auscultation over the lungs multiple bruits could be heard. His observations were normal and proctoscopy didn't reveal any haemorrhoids. What is the most likely diagnosis?

A. Haemophilia A
B. Angiodysplasia
C. Peutz-Jeghers sydnrome
D. Meckel's diverticulum
E. Hereditary haemorrhagic telangiectasia (HHT)

19. A patient with long-term liver cirrhosis secondary to alcoholic hepatitis presents to hospital with acute oliguria and worsening ascites. His blood tests reveal a rise in urea and creatinine. As part of the investigations a renal biopsy is taken, and shows a normal renal histology. Which of the following is most likely to be part of this patient's treatment plan?

A. Captopril
B. Intravenous Hartmann's
C. Prednisolone and cyclophosphamide
D. Terlipressin
E. Plasma exchange

20. A patient presents to hospital with abdominal distension. On examination it is deemed that the distension is due to ascites. An ascitic tap is taken and the fluid analysed:

Neutrophils: 30 cells per mm^3

Which of the following medications should be started?

A. Cefotaxime
B. Ciprofloxacin
C. Furosemide
D. Bendrofluromethiazide
E. Spironolactone

21. An elderly lady has dysphagia, regurgitation of food and severe halitosis. On examination she is found to have a small round fluctuant mass in the left anterior triangle of the neck. Which is the single most appropriate investigation to confirm the diagnosis?

A. Barium swallow
B. Cervical X-ray
C. Magnetic-resonance imaging (MRI) of the neck
D. Ultrasound and fine needle aspiration
E. Oesophagoscopy

22. A patient known to have liver cirrhosis as a result of a chronic hepatitis B infection presents to hospital with haematemisis. He is treated with intravenous terlipressin and an endoscopy is carried out along with variceal banding. The patient is due to be discharged, which of the following medications should be prescribed as prophylaxis to prevent a further gastrointestinal bleed?

A. Omeprazole
B. Amlodipine
C. Propranolol
D. Tranexamic acid
E. Desmopressin

23. A 40-year-old male presents to his doctor with long standing dyspepsia. He described having epigastric pain that is worse at night and before meals. On further questioning he mentioned that his stools have become a dark black colour recently. Which of the following is the most appropriate next step in this patient's management?

A. Lifestyle changes and review in 4 weeks
B. Trial of Lansoprazole
C. Trial of magnesium trisilicate
D. Helicobacter pylori breath test
E. Oesophagogastroduodenoscopy (OGD)

24. A 50-year-old man with a history of gastric carcinoma presents 1 year after a gastrectomy with pins and needles in his feet. Which of the following should be given to treat his symptoms?

A. Advice on alcohol intake
B. Oral vitamin B co-strong
C. Intramuscular hydroxocobalamin
D. Metformin
E. Duloxetine

25. A young patient is being investigated for inflammatory bowel disease, and a faecal calprotectin is requested. Which of the following medications can cause a raised faecal calprotectin?

A. Paracetamol
B. Naproxen
C. Tramadol
D. Hydorxychloroquie
E. Prednisolone

26. A 55-year-old male with primary sclerosing cholangitis is being considered for a liver transplant. Which of the following features is most likely to be an indication for the procedure?

A. Raised immunoglobulins
B. Presence of caput medusae
C. Concurrent ulcerative colitis
D. Raised transaminases
E. Presence of shifting dullness on examination

27. Following an endoscopy a patient is diagnosed with gastric mucosal associated lymphoid tissue (MALT) lymphoma. He also has a positive ^{13}C urea breath test. Which of the following is the most appropriate first line treatment regime?

A. Amoxicillin, clarithromycin and omeprazole
B. Radiotherapy
C. Chemotherapy
D. Surgical removal
E. Sclerotherapy

28. A 23-year-old male is admitted to hospital following a first flare of Crohn's disease. His symptoms are now under control. He is currently on a reducing dose of steroids. Which of the following drugs is the most appropriate first line medication to maintain remission?

A. Azathioprine
B. Methotrexate
C. Ciclosporin
D. Infliximab
E. Sulfasalazine

29. A 55-year-old farmer presents with reduced consciousness, urinary and faecal incontinence. He has severe watery diarrhoea and is sweating profusely. On examination his heart rate is 65 beats per minute (bpm), he is normotensive and his pupils are constricted. Which of the following drugs should be administered?

A. Adrenaline
B. Naloxone
C. Loperamide
D. Pralidoxime
E. Haloperidol

30. An elderly man presents to hospital following two episodes of heavy haematemesis and is haemodynamically unstable. His only significant past medical history is an abdominal aortic aneurysm that was repaired two years ago. Which of the following is the most likely underlying cause of his symptoms?

A. Angiodysplasia
B. Mesenteric ischaemia
C. Dieulafoy lesion
D. Aorto-enteric fistula
E. Ruptured oesophageal varices

31. A patient has taken an overdose of an unknown substance 12 hours ago. She presents with severe abdominal pain, haematemisis and maleana. She is tachycardic and hypotensive. An abdominal X-ray shows multiple well-defined round opaque lesions in the gut. Which of the following should be given?

A. Activated charcoal
B. N-acetylcysteine
C. Sodium bicarbonate
D. Desferrioxamine
E. Ethylenediaminetetraacetic acid (EDTA)

Gastrointestinal Answers

1. B
Interferon gamma release assay test and chest X-ray

Infliximab is a tumour necrosis factor (TNFα) inhibitor, which can reactivate latent tuberculosis (TB); therefore before starting infliximab all patients should be screened for TB. The interferon gamma release assay is able to test for latent TB and the chest X-ray is also useful to look for apical scaring, which could also indicate a latent TB infection. This is the most accurate way of screening patients.

The mantoux test is unable to differentiate between latent TB and previous TB infections, so it is less useful. Also it is known to give false positive results if patients have been infected with other forms of mycobacterium or had a previous Bacillus Calmette-Guérin (BCG) vaccination.

Sputum cultures would be used to diagnose active TB. As far as we know this patient is asymptomatic and therefore unlikely to have active TB. The lack of a productive cough means sputum cultures would not be an option anyway.

Blood tests for liver and renal function are sometimes required before starting drugs, but the main concern is that infliximab may reactivate latent TB.

Nerve conduction studies may be required if a patient was taking a medication known to cause a peripheral neuropathy, but this is not a concern when using infliximab.

2. A
Acute pancreatitis

This patient has presented with epigastric pain, vomiting and steator-rhea. The acute pancreatitis has been caused by a combination of drugs (mesalazine, azathioprine and steroids) that this patient is currently taking. Other drug causes of pancreatitis include alcohol, sodium valproate and diuretics.

A leaking abdominal aortic aneurysm wouldn't have lasted for 3 days and would have caused a reduced haemoglobin level.

Addison's disease would cause hyponatraemia, hyperkalaemia, and hypoglycemia, which are not present in the current blood test results.

A perforated duodenal ulcer would have caused reduced haemoglobin and raised urea, melaena and hypovlaemic shock. This patient would have presented much earlier.

An inferior myocardial infarction could cause epigastric pain, but wouldn't have caused diarrhoea. Also it would be extremely rare for a 30 year old to have a myocardial infarction.

3. D
Flucloxacillin

This gentleman has developed cholestatic jaundice, which is a recognised side effect of flucloxacillin and often develops a short period after the antibiotic course has been completed. This presents with jaundice, puritis, pale stools and dark urine.

Erythromycin is a macrolide antibiotic, which can cause hepatitis, however this would occur while the patient is taking the antibiotic, not once it had stopped. Also it doesn't cause cholestasis and therefore wouldn't present with pale stools.

Clindamycin is a broad-spectrum antibiotic, which increases the risk of Clostridium difficile infections. It can be used to treat Staphylococcal infections in patients with penicillin allergies and therefore can be used to treat cellulitis, but given the risk of Clostridium difficile infections it is not first-line therapy.

Phenoxymethylpenicillin is also known as penicillin V, and can be added to flucloxacillin to treat cellulitis infections if there is a concern that the underlying cause may be a Streptococcus rather than a Staphylococcus.

Trimethoprim is used to treat urinary tract infections, and it can rarely cause a megaloblastic anaemia and bone marrow suppression because of its inhibition of folate activity.

4. B
Positive anti-smooth muscle antibody

This patient has developed autoimmune hepatitis. This is often associated with other autoimmune conditions such as pernicious anaemia, autoimmune thyroiditis and type 1 diabetes mellitus. It can present with fever, puritis, amenorrhoea and polyarthralgia. The liver screen would show a raised anti-nuclear antibody (ANA), anti-smooth muscle antibody, and raised IgG in autoimmune hepatitis type 1. Other less common antibodies found include anti-liver/kidney microsomal type 1 (LKM1) antibody in type 2, and antibodies against soluble liver antigen or liver-pancreas antigen in type 3.

A raised IgM can be found in primary biliary cirrhosis. This often affects females of a slightly older age range. It causes xanthelasma and xanthemata, and it also causes malabsorption of the fat soluble vitamins.

Alpha-fetoprotein is a tumour marker for hepatocellular carcinoma. Risk factors for this would include cirrhosis, especially if caused by hepatitis viruses B and C. It is likely to cause weight loss and right upper quadrant pain.

Raised ferritin can be found in many inflammatory conditions, as it is an acute phase protein. However here it is referring to hereditary haemochromatosis, which is an autosomal recessive condition that leads to excessive hepatic iron storage. It can present with polyarthralgia, skin pigmentation and polyuria and polydipsia due to development of diabetes mellitus.

5. C
Colestyramine

Colestyramine is a bile acid sequestrant and it prevents reabsorption of bile acids, thus reducing jaundice and puritis. However it also causes reduced absorption of fat soluble vitamins. This woman has become vitamin D deficient and developed osteomalacia. This is also likely to be exacerbated by her liver cirrhosis, as the liver is required to convert cholecalciferol to calcidiol. Osteomalacia often causes bone pain and can lead to a proximal myopathy, hence the waddling gait. Her blood results also indicate osteomalacia.

Naltrexone is an opioid antagonist and is often used in treating alcohol dependence.

Codeine phosphate is an opiate used to treat pain. Its side effects include puritis, nausea and vomiting and also constipation. It should be avoided in liver cirrhosis as constipation can lead to hepatic encephalopathy.

Ursodeoxycholic acid is used in treatment of primary biliary cirrhosis. It is thought to normalise the liver function tests (LFTs) but doesn't have much impact on long-term prognosis.

Acamprosate is used in treatment of alcohol dependence and is thought to reduce cravings. It's side effects include weight gain and low libido.

6. D
Liver biopsy with pearl stain

This patient has hereditary haemochromatosis, which is a genetic condition caused by a recessive mutation in the HFE gene on chromosome 6. It leads to iron deposition in the liver causing liver failure, pancreas causing bronze diabetes, pituitary gland causing hypogonadism, and heart causing a dilated cardiomyopathy. It is also associated with chondrocalcinosis, which causes polyarthralgia. The definitive diagnostic test is a liver biopsy with a pearl stain, which stains for iron. Serum ferritin would be raised, but this can also be raised in inflammatory conditions, as it is an acute phase protein. It is not specific to haemochromatosis.

> Periodic acid–Schiff (PAS) stain can be used to diagnose α_1-antitrypsin deficiency, which can also cause liver cirrhosis but also affects the lungs causing emphysema.
>
> Short synathen test is used to diagnose Addison's disease. Synthetic adrenocorticotrophin (ACTH) is injected and cortisol levels are measured. In Addison's disease the cortisol remains low. It can present non specifically with nausea and vomiting, abdominal pain, hyperpigmentation and polyuria and polydipsia.
>
> Fasting venous glucose can diagnose diabetes mellitus, which may present with polyuria and polydipsia. In this case it is likely to be raised due to the presence of 'bronze' diabetes.

7. A
Pseudomembranous colitis

This patient has developed a Clostridium difficile infection as a result of using broad-spectrum antibiotics. C.difficile can be present in the normal flora of the gut, but when broad-spectrum antibiotics are used they lead to death of the other normal flora and overgrowth of C.difficile. It produces toxins A and B, which lead to a psuedomembrnous colitis, which is the presence of yellow adherent plaques on an inflamed mucosa. The worst culprits for causing a C.difficile infection are cephalosporins, clindamycin and ciprofloxacin.

Cobble stoning and serosal fat wrapping are both found in Crohn's disease, which is inflammatory bowel disease caused by transmural inflammation of the gut.

Pseudopolyposis is found in ulcerative colitis, which is an inflammatory bowel disease caused by inflammation of the lamina propria of the colon.

Colonic fibrosis can occur following long-term inflammation and also after radiotherapy.

8. B
Granulomas around the bile ducts

This patient has developed primary biliary cirrhosis. This is caused by interlobular bile ducts being damaged by granulomatous inflammation. This results in a cholestatic jaundice, cirrhosis and portal hypertension. Patients can be asymptomatic or present with puritis as a result of jaundice. It also causes malabsorption of fat soluble vitamins, xanthelasma and xanthemata. It is also associated with autoimmune thyroid disease and Sjrogen's syndrome.

Fibrous obliterative cholangitis is found in primary sclerosing cholangitis. This condition is associated with ulcerative colitis and leads to autoimmune destruction of both the intra and extra hepatic bile ducts. It also causes cholestatic jaundice.

Ground glass hepatocytes occur in a chronic hepatitis B infection, and are a histological finding seen upon liver biopsy.

Interface hepatitis is where the inflammatory cells spill out from the portal tracts. This can occur in autoimmune hepatitis. Other histological findings would include piecemeal necrosis.

Steatohepatitis is where there is fat deposition in the hepatocytes. This occurs most commonly in alcoholic liver disease and non-alcoholic steatohepatitis (NASH).

9. C
Corkscrew oesophagus

This patient has developed oesophageal spasm. This presents with intermittent dysphagia and can also cause cardiac sounding chest pain. It is relieved by muscle relaxants such as nitrates, calcium channel blockers and sildenafil. However unlike cardiac chest pain, which can be relived within seconds, nitrates take longer to relieve oesophageal spasm. A barium swallow can be used in the diagnosis and shows abnormal oesophageal contractions such as the cork screw appearance.

The dilated tapering oesophagus and bird beak appearance can occur in achalasia. Achalasia is where the lower oesophageal sphincter is unable to relax due to damage to the myenteric plexus. It presents with sudden onset dysphagia affecting both liquids and solids.

Zenker's diverticulum is also known as a pharyngeal pouch, and is where the pharyngeal wall balloons outwards. It presents with dysphagia, regurgitation of food and severe halitosis. There is often a visible bulge in the side of the neck.

Hiatus hernia is where the stomach protrudes through the hiatus present in the diaphram. This can present as either a sliding hernia, which traces straight upward, or a rolling hernia where the side of the stomach protrudes. Rolling hernias are at risk of strangulation and ischaemia; and therefore require surgery. Whereas sliding hernias do not and can be treated medically. Patients with a hiatus hernia develop gastro-oesophageal reflux and complain of heartburn (which can progress to oesophagitis and odynophagia), water brash, and a hoarse voice due to laryngitis.

10. E
Nicorandil

This gentleman was prescribed nicorandil as an antianginal medication. Nicorandil has a vasodilatory effect similar to that of nitrates, but it is not frequently prescribed because one of its side effects is severe mucosal ulceration, which can lead to gastrointestinal ulcers and may progress to perforation. It can also cause skin and eye ulceration.

Atorvastatin is a statin and acts by HMG-CoA reductase inhibition to reduce cholesterol production. Its main side effects are myalgia and hepatitis.

Bisoprolol and diltiazem both act on the atrioventricular node to reduce the heart rate, and therefore can both cause bradycardia.

Clopidogrel is an antiplatelet medication, which can increase the risk of bleeding, but wouldn't cause the florid ulceration that is seen with nicorandil.

11. B
Insertion of a nasogastric tube and intravenous 0.9% saline

This patient has developed acute pancreatitis secondary to an ERCP. The management of this is mainly conservative. Patients are given lots of intravenous fluids due to lots of third space losses and are made 'nil by mouth' in an attempt to allow the pancreas to rest and recover. Morphine is often required for analgesia. Patients require intense monitoring for any complications such as shock, acute respiratory distress syndrome (ARDS), acute kidney injury (AKI), sepsis, hypocalcaemia and hyperglycemia.

Cefuroxime and metronidazole is an antibiotic regime used to cover infections caused by flora of the intestines. It can be given prophylactically prior to surgery or as treatment for diverticulitis and other intestinal infections.

Domperidone is an antiemetic and diclofenac is a non-steroidal anti-inflammatory drug (NSAID), both may help with the symptoms being described, but are not used in pancreatitis and are not part of the definitive management.

A cholecystectomy would be used to treat gallstones. It often occurs as an elective operation a few weeks after acute cholecystitis to allow the inflammation to settle.

An emergency laparotomy would be required if this patient had a perforation.

12. B
Melanosis coli

This is a form of microscopic colitis, which is caused by laxative abuse, most commonly due to senna. Microscopic colitis presents with watery diarrhoea, a normal colonoscopy and characteristic histology. In melanosis coli there is brown pigmentation in the macrophages in the lamina propria (also known as lipofuscin-laden macrophages). This patient is likely to be suffering from anorexia nervosa. She has a low body mass index (BMI) and as result developed amenorrhea. Patients with this condition may use laxatives to aid weight loss.

Lymphocytic colitis is another type of microscopic colitis and histology shows lymphocytes in the colonic epithelium.

Whipple's disease is caused by Tropheryma whipplei and is a rare condition that most commonly affects middle aged Caucasian males. It presents with arthralgia and malabsorption (causing diarrhea, weight loss and abdominal pain). It progresses to cause reversible dementia, facial myoclonus and systemic symptoms of fever, night sweats and lymphadenopathy. It is diagnosed by a jejunal biopsy showing macrophages with granules that stain positive for periodic acid–Schiff (PAS).

Entamoeba histolytica is a protozoon that invades the bowel and causes flask shaped ulcers in the colon, resulting in bloody diarrhoea. It can also spread to the liver resulting in a liver abscess, which presents with a swinging fever, right upper quadrant pain, tenderness and hepatomegaly.

13. D
Cholangiocarcinoma

This patient has an obstructive jaundice. Conjugated bilirubin is soluble and therefore can be excreted in the urine; this is raised. Urobilinogen is formed by bacteria in the small intestine, which convert conjugated bilirubin to urobilinogen. This is then reabsorbed and excreted by the kidneys. If this is absent it means that conjugated bilirubin is not being allowed to enter the small intestine. Cholangiocarcinoma is the only cause of obstructive jaundice listed. It is a biliary tree malignancy associated with liver flukes and primary sclerosing cholangitis (PSC). It presents with weight loss, abdominal pain and obstructive jaundice.

Budd-Chiari syndrome is hepatic vein obstruction due to thrombosis or tumour. This causes hepatic ischaemia and damage to the hepatocytes. It presents with right upper quadrant pain, hepatomegaly and ascites.

Budd-Chiari syndrome, hepatocellular carcinoma and statin induced hepatitis all cause a hepatic jaundice, and therefore would still have urobilinogen present in the urine.

Gilbert's syndrome is a genetic condition that results in reduced levels of glucuronyl transferase (the enzyme used to conjugate bilirubin). It causes a raised unconjugated bilirubin especially if patients have an infection. It is often asymptomatic and none of the other liver function tests (LFTs) are affected.

14. B
Tissue transglutaminase antibody

This patient has coeliac disease, which is an autoimmune disease, whereby a reaction to gluten in the diet and leads to villous atrophy within the small intestine. This causes malabsorption leading to weight loss, diarrhoea, steatorrhea (which is described above as offensive smelling stools that don't flush), bloating and abdominal pain. This patient has also developed a normocytic anaemia as a result of a combined iron and folate deficiency. Antibodies that can be tested for include tissue transglutaminase antibody (most sensitive), anti-endomysial antibody (most specific) and anti-gliadin (not commonly used). Therefore tissue transglutaminase antibody is used as a screening test, and anti-endomysial antibody is used to confirm the diagnosis. Despite this a duodenal biopsy is still the gold standard for diagnosis.

P-ANCA is often positive in ulcerative colitis, and ASCA is found in Crohn's disease. These are both forms of inflammatory bowel disease and therefore would have caused diarrhoea with both mucus and blood present.

15. E
Labetalol

This patient has acute intermittent porphyria. This is caused by an accumulation of porphyrins. During attacks the urinary prophobilinogens are raised but faecal prophyrins remain normal. Many things including infections and drugs can trigger attacks. It classically presents with abdominal pain, neurological symptoms, hypertension and tachycardia due to sympathetic overdrive. Other features include a fever and hyponatraemia. Treatment is intravenous fluids, carbohydrates, and haematin to inhibit production of porphyrinogen precursors. During acute intermittent porphyria only beta-blockers are safe to lower blood pressure. All other antihypertensives can exacerbate the attack.

16. D
Dapsone

This patient has developed dermatitis herpetiformis as a result of underlying coeliac disease. This can be treated with dapsone. The patient must still adhere to a gluten free diet.

17. C
Ultrasound scan of the abdomen

This patient has Budd-Chiari syndrome, which is hepatic vein obstruction either by a thrombus or tumour. It causes hepatic ischaemia and presents with liver failure. It causes hepatomegaly, ascites and abdominal pain. Diagnosis can be made by ultrasound, computed tomography (CT) or magnetic resonance imaging (MRI). In the acute setting the underlying cause should be treated. If the condition is chronic then a liver transplant may be required. This patient has had multiple deep vein thrombosis and therefore is likely to have an underlying coagulopathy and be at risk of further blood clots.

A toxicology screen would be useful if this patient had a suspected paracetamol overdose. This could present in a very non-specific manner. Symptoms would include nausea, vomiting and right upper quadrant pain. Treatment would include N-acetylcysteine. If not treated in time it could then progress to cause fulminant liver failure with jaundice and hepatic encephalopathy, which would require a liver transplant. Paracetamol overdose is unlikely in this patient due to the presence of ascites, which suggests portal hypertension.

Intravenous cefuroxime and metronidazole an antibiotic regime used to cover infections caused by flora of the intestines. It can be given prophylactically prior to surgery or as treatment for diverticulitis and other intestinal infections.

18. E
Hereditary haemorrhagic telangiectasia (HHT)

This is also known as Osler-Weber-Rendu syndrome. It is an auto-somal dominant condition that results in abnormal blood vessel formation. Its features include telangiectasia on the lips, arterio-venous malformations (especially in the lungs), and recurrent epistaxis. It can also affect the bowel causing gastrointestinal bleeds. The bruits heard over this patient's lungs have been caused by multiple arteriovenous malformations.

Haemophilia A is an X-linked recessive disorder, causing a lack of clotting factor VIII. It causes severe bleeding; especially following injury, and can result in haemoarthrosis and haematomas. It could also cause gastrointestinal bleeds and epistaxis, but wouldn't cause the arteriovenous malformations seen in this patient.

Angiodysplasia describes small vascular malformations that are found in the gut. It can affect the upper and lower gastrointestinal tract and bleeding is often intermittent. It typically occurs in the elderly and can be associated with aortic stenosis in what is known as Heyde's syndrome. Active lesions can most accurately be diag-nosed using a 99 mLc radionuclide-labelled red-cell imaging. This condition would cause rectal bleeding but not epistaxis.

Meckel's diverticulum is a bulge in the wall of the small intes-tine that occurs 2 feet away from the ileocaecal valve, is often 2 inches in length and affects 2% of the population. It can contain ectopic gastric and pancreatic tissue. It is often asymptomatic but can cause rectal bleeding, or obstruction due to intussusception or volvulus. Treatment involves surgical removal. In cases of acute abdomen where surgery is indicated (such as in appendicitis), sur-geons often search for and remove a Meckel's diverticulum to prevent future complications.

19. D
Terlipressin

This patient has developed hepatorenal syndrome as a result of chronic liver disease. This is caused by portal hypertension leading to release of splanchnic vasodilators. This results in arterial vasodilation and a reduced circulating volume; there is also renal vasoconstriction, which causes pre-renal failure. There are two types of hepatorenal syndrome. Type 1 is rapidly progressive and has a median survival of less than two weeks. Type 2 has a more steady deterioration. They present with a rising creatinine, hyponatraemia and normal renal histology. Treatment involves using intravenous albumin to restore the circulating volume and splanchnic vasoconstrictors such as terlipressin.

Captopril is an angiotensin converting enzyme (ACE) inhibitor and wouldn't be given to anyone with acute deterioration of his or her renal function, as it causes dilation of the post-glomerular arteriole, thus further reducing the glomerular filtration rate (GFR).

Prednisolone and cyclophosphamide is an immunosuppressant regime used to treat autoimmune conditions such as granulomatosis with polyangiitis (otherwise known as Wegener's granulomatosis). If this fails treatment may be stepped up to include plasma exchange. Granulomatosis with polyangiitis causes a rapidly progressive glomerulonephritis and therefore would show crescentic glomerulonephritis on the renal biopsy.

Intravenous Hartmann's is not given in patients with liver cirrhosis as they are unable to metabolise the lactate and its use can lead to a metabolic lactic acidosis.

20. E
Spironolactone

The ascitic fluid has a low level of neutrophils and therefore a spontaneous bacterial peritonitis is unlikely and this patient just has uncomplicated ascites. If neutrophils >250 cells per mm^3 then a spontaneous bacterial peritonitis would be suspected, and cefotaxime should be given. Ciprofloxacin can be used as long-term prophylaxis against spontaneous bacterial peritonitis, and should be considered especially in patients with a raised international normal-ised ratio (INR), low serum albumin and low ascitic albumin.

Spironolactone is an aldosterone antagonist. In liver cirrhosis there is increased pooling of blood in the splanchnic system and therefore a reduced blood flow to the kidneys. This in turn activates the renin-angiotensin system causing salt and fluid retention. Spironolactone acts against aldosterone and reduces salt and fluid retention and therefore is the first line treatment for ascites.

Furosemide, which is a loop diuretic, can be added if the response is poor.

Bendroflumethiazide is a thiazide diuretic, and has no role in treating ascites.

21. A
Barium swallow

This patient has a pharyngeal pouch (also known as a Zenker's diverticu-lum) and is where the pharyngeal wall balloons outwards causing dyspha-gia, regurgitation of food and severe halitosis. A barium swallow is also used to diagnose achalasia.

Cervical X-ray would be used if any fractures were suspected in the cervical spine.

MRI of the neck may be used if malignancy was suspected. It can give more detailed imaging of the larynx and pharynx.

Ultrasound and fine needle aspiration would also be used to diagnose malignancy, for example if a lymphoma was suspected.

Oesophagoscopy would be used to directly look at the oesophagus and therefore is used to diagnose conditions such as Barrett's oesophagus, or oesophageal cancer.

22. C
Propranolol

This patient has developed oesophageal varices due to his cirrhosis causing portal hypertension and increased blood flow through the splanchnic system. There is increased collateral blood flow through the portosystemic anastomosis. These are present around the lower oesophagus, in the stomach around the umbilicus (known as caput medusae) and in the rectum. This high pressure flow through a low pressure system, and along with a coagulopathy due to liver failure, and thrombocytopenia due to functional hypersplenism leads these areas being prone to bleeding. Acutely terlipressin (a vasopressin analogue) is used to cause splanchnic vasoconstriction, and endoscopic banding is used as definitive management. Propranolol is a non-specific beta-blocker and acts to cause vasodilation of the splanchnic veins, thus reducing the pressure and reducing the risk of bleeding in the future. Therefore it can be given as prophylaxis.

Omeprazole is a proton pump inhibitor, and could be used to treat and prevent peptic ulcers.

Amlodipine is a dihydropyridine calcium channel blocker used to treat hypertension, but has no role in treating varices.

Tranexamic acid inhibits the breakdown of fibrin in blood clots. It can be given to treat menorrhagia, and other bleeding disorders.

Desmopressin is another vasopressin analogue. It can be given as a nasal spray to treat haemophilia A and von Willebrand syndrome. It acts to cause vasoconstriction and also increases release of factor VIII from the endothelium of the blood vessels. It is useful in minor bleeds caused by these conditions but has no role in treating varices.

23. E
Oesophagogastroduodenoscopy (OGD)

This patient is describing dyspepsia and melaena (which is one of the red flag symptoms). Other red flag symptoms include; new onset dyspepsia in a patient over 55 years old, anaemia, weight loss, anorexia, haematemesis, dysphagia and recent onset of progressive symptoms. If any of these are present patients require an upper gastrointestinal endoscopy.

If none of these are present then patients are first advised to make lifestyle changes (such as weight loss, avoiding alcohol and spicy foods, and not eating big meals before bedtime). The general practitioner (GP) will also review any drugs that may be causing their symptoms such as non-steroidal anti-inflammatory drugs (NSAIDs), and prescribe an antacid such as magnesium trisilicate for four weeks.

If the patient is reviewed and still complains of symptoms following these changes then they should be tested for Helicobacter pylori. The breath test is most commonly used. If positive then patients are treated with triple therapy and then re-tested. If negative then patients are given a 4 week trial of proton pump inhibitors such as lansoprazole.

24. C
Intramuscular hydroxocobalamin

This patient has developed a peripheral neuropathy due to vitamin B12 deficiency following his gastrectomy. Vitamin B12 absorption occurs in the terminal ileum. However to be absorbed it must be bound to intrinsic factor which is released by the parietal cells in the stomach. Without intrinsic factor it cannot be absorbed, therefore the supplements must be given as an intramuscular injection.

Vitamin B-Co strong is a multivitamin with contains a combination of the B vitamins. It is often given to alcoholics, who are at risk of developing a thiamine (vitamin B1) deficiency.

Alcohol can also lead to a peripheral neuropathy but this is not the cause in this patient.

Metformin is a biguanide used to treat type 2 diabetes.

Duloxetine is a serotonin-norepinephrine reuptake inhibitor (SNRI), which can be used to treat a peripheral neuropathy in diabetes.

25. B
Naproxen

Calprotectin is secreted by neutrophils and is a marker of inflammation. Faecal calprotectin is used as a biomarker for intestinal inflammation and can be raised in inflammatory bowel disease, gastrointestinal infections and malignancy. Naproxen is a non-steroidal anti-inflammatory drug (NSAID), and all drugs in this class can also increase the faecal calprotectin. NSAIDs are also contraindicated in inflammatory bowel disease because they can exacerbate the disease.

26. E
Presence of shifting dullness on examination

When considering patients for a liver transplant it is important to access the synthetic function of the liver. If this is compromised it causes raised bilirubin (jaundice), raised international normalised ratio (INR) (coagulopathy), reduced albumin (ascites) and raised nitrogenous waste (hepatic encephalopathy and asterixis). These are the five signs of decompensated liver failure. Shifting dullness on examination is a sign of ascites, which occurs in decompensated liver failure and therefore is a true indication of liver damage.

Immunoglobulins and P-ANCA levels may be used to monitor the effectiveness of treatment, but don't give any indication of how severe the liver damage is.

Transaminases (ALT and AST) are present in the liver function tests (LFTs), and are released when hepatocytes are damaged but don't give a true indication of liver function.

Ulcerative colitis is a risk factor for developing primary sclerosing cholangitis but is not an indication of how severe the liver disease is.

Caput medusae are dilated epigastric veins and form as a result of portal hypertension causing portosystemic shunts. It is often seen in severe liver cirrhosis, but isn't a marker used to grade liver damage.

27. A
Amoxicillin, clarithromycin and ompeprazole

Mucosal associated lymphoid tissue (MALT) lymphoma is a B-cell lymphoma that arises from the marginal zone of the MALT. It is almost always associated with an underlying Helicobacter pylori infection. Treatment of the underlying infection is often enough to eradicate the MALT lymphoma.

This patient has had a positive ^{13}C urea breath test, which is used to identify a Helicobacter pylori infection. Therefore he should be started on triple therapy (amoxicillin, clarithromycin and a proton pump inhibitor).

Radiotherapy and chemotherapy are reserved for the rare cases that are not associated with an underlying infection. Surgical removal and sclerotherapy don't have a role in treatment.

28. A
Azathioprine

The first line treatment for maintaining remission in Crohn's disease is azathioprine. It is a useful steroid sparing agent. Methotrexate is only used if azathioprine doesn't have a desired affect. Ciclosporin is another second line drug. It is more commonly used in ulcerative colitis to treat severe acute flares. Infliximab is the last line of medication. It is used in severe acute flares, perianal disease and also in patients who's condition cannot be controlled by any other medication. Sulfasalazine efficacy in Crohn's disease is unproven, but it may be trialed in some patients. It is more commonly used in ulcerative colitis.

29. D
Pralidoxime

This patient has organophosphate insecticide poisoning. Organophosphates act by inhibiting the acetylcholinesterase in the nerve synapses, which results in parasympathetic over activation. It presents with salivation, lacrimation, urinary incontinence, diarrhoea, bradycardia, pupillary constriction and confusion. Treatment involves washing the skin, giving atropine (a muscarinic antagonist) and pralidoxime. Pralidoxime is an oxide compound, which binds non-competitively to the acetlycholineserase enzyme, and then binds to the organophosphate. This changes its shape so it can no longer bind to the acetylcholinesterase enzyme. The conjoined pralidoxime/organophosphate compound unbinds from the site, thus allowing the enzyme to function again. Diazepam may also be given to prevent seizures.

Adrenaline is not likely to be required, but may be needed if patients become severely bradycardic and the above medications are not working.

Naloxone is an opiate receptor antagonist, which is given in opiate overdoses.

Loperamide is an opiate receptor agonist that binds to the myenteric plexus in the large intestine and decreases the smooth muscle activity. It is used to treat diarrhoea.

Haloperidol is a typical antipsychotic drug, which is used to treat psychosis, to sedate patients and also as an antiemetic in palliative care.

30. D
Aorto-enteric fistula

Any patient who presents with signs of an upper gastrointestinal bleed and has had a previous aortic graft repair must be considered to have an aorto-enteric fistula until proven otherwise. They would be investigated by use of a computed tomography (CT) scan and endoscopy. It can present with a minor bleed, which may rapidly progress to life threatening blood loss.

Angiodysplasia describes small vascular malformations that are found in the gut. It can affect the upper and lower gastrointestinal tract and bleeding is often intermittent. It typically occurs in the elderly and can be associated with aortic stenosis in what is known as Heyde's syndrome.

Thrombosis or embolism in the mesenteric arteries or mesenteric vein thrombosis causes mesenteric ischaemia. It should be suspected in any patient presenting with abdominal pain and atrial fibrillation. It causes severe abdominal pain, a rising lactate and hypovolaemia, and leads to shock.

Dieulafoy lesion is a large tortuous arteriole present in the submucosa of the stomach, which is prone to rupture and bleeding. It is a relatively rare cause of upper gastrointestinal bleeding.

31. D
Desferrioxamine

This patient has overdosed on iron tablets, and developed acute iron poisoning. This presents with abdominal pain and upper gastrointestinal bleeding. The abdominal X-ray can identify the iron tablets, because metals show up as being opaque on radiographs. Treatment involves using desferrioxamine, which is an iron chelator.

Activated charcoal is commonly used in poisoning, but can only be used up to one hour after the overdose has been ingested.

N-acetylcysteine is used to treat a paracetamol overdose. This would often present with non-specific symptoms such as abdominal pain and vomiting. It then progresses to jaundice and encephalopathy as a result of liver damage.

Sodium bicarbonate is administered in an aspirin overdose to aid the excretion of aspirin. Aspirin overdose would present with nausea, vomiting, hyperventilation, tinnitus, vertigo and can progress to cause seizures.

Ethylenediaminetetraacetic acid (EDTA) is given to treat lead poisoning. In the acute setting this may also present with abdominal pain, vomiting and diarrhoea. It also causes muscle weakness, paraesthesia and intravascular haemolysis which presents with haematuria.

Haematology Questions

1. A 34-year-old vegetarian woman with well-controlled hypothyroidism is found to be anaemic during a routine check up. She is treated with a new medication. A month later she presents with weight gain, fatigue, dry skin and menorrhagia. Which medication was used to treat her anaemia?

A. Ferrous sulphate
B. Folic acid
C. Oral vitamin B12
D. Intramuscular hydroxocobalamin
E. Erythropoietin

2. A patient with a background of atrial fibrillation and a previous ischaemic stroke was recently started on rivaroxaban for anticoagulation. Which of the following blood tests should be monitored regularly?

A. International normalised ratio (INR)
B. Activated partial thromboplastin time (APTT) ratio
C. Full blood count
D. Urea and creatinine
E. Total cholestrol

3. An elderly woman presents to her doctor following excessive bleeding after a dental operation. His blood tests show the following:

Haemoglobin:	125 g/L
Platelet count:	356×10^9 /L
Prothrombin time (PT):	13 seconds
Activated partial thromboplastin time (APTT):	103 seconds
APTT after 50/50 mix with normal plasma:	103 seconds

Which of the following is the most likely underlying diagnosis?

A. Haemophilia A
B. Acquired haemophilia
C. Von Willebrand's disease
D. Antiphospholipid syndrome
E. Vitamin K deficiency

4. An elderly patient is found to have a raised white blood cell count during a routine blood test. The doctor suspects this patient may have chronic myeloid leukaemia. Which of the following findings would increase the likelihood of this suspicion?

A. Presence of a JAK2 mutation
B. Right shift seen on a blood film
C. Cervical lymphadenopathy
D. Reduced neutrophil alkaline phosphatase
E. Lymphocytosis

5. A young female patient presents to her doctor with easy bruising and a purpuric rash. She also reports bleeding from her gums when she is brushing her teeth. Her initial blood tests show a platelet count of 5×10^9 per litre, but an otherwise normal full blood count and normal renal function. Which of the following is the most likely underlying diagnosis?

A. Idiopathic thrombocytopenic purpura (ITP)
B. Thrombotic thrombocytopenic purpura (TTP)
C. Meningococcal septicaemia
D. Haemophilia A
E. Liver cirrhosis

6. A patent with a history of chronic kidney disease is started on heparin for thromboembolism prophylaxis. One week later this patient develops a deep vein thrombosis in his left calf. His blood tests show he is thrombocytopenic. Which of the following is most likely to be part of this patient's treatment?

A. Platelet transfusion
B. Protamine sulphate
C. Dalteparin and warfarin
D. Danaparoid or lepirudin
E. Aspirin

7. Which of the following is not a side effect of heparin?

A. Thrombocytopenia
B. Osteoporosis
C. Haemorrhage
D. Hypokalaemia
E. Urticaria

8. A 32-year-old Greek male has a routine blood test at his general practitioner (GP) surgery. The results are as follows:

Haemglobin: 95 g/L
Mean corpusclar volume (MCV):   64 fL

The iron studies were normal. As a result the doctor ordered haemo-globin electrophoresis and a blood film. Which of the following results is most likely to be found?

A. Absent HbA
B. Raised HbA_2
C. Normal HbF
D. Polychromasia
E. Pappenheimer bodies

9. Following a bone marrow transplant a patient is immunosuppressed-with ciclosporin. He is started on a new drug, which results in him devel-oping oliguria, and bilateral pitting oedema. On examination he is found to have a hypertension and a course tremor. His blood tests show an increase in serum creatinine. Which of the following new drugs may this patient have been started on?

A. Erythromycin
B. Griseofulvin
C. Phenytoin
B. Carbamazepine
E. Gliclazide

10. A patient with known essential thrombocythaemia presents to his doctor following six months of weight loss, fevers and night sweats. On examination he is found to have massive hepatosplenomegaly. The doctor orders some investigations. Which of the following is most likely to be found on the blood film?

A. Auer rods
B. Mirror cells
C. Leukoerythroblastic cells
D. Rouleaux formation
E. Left shift

11. A 22-year-old male presents with fevers, night sweats and weight loss. He is subsequently diagnosed with Hodgkin's lymphoma. As part of his investigations a chest X-ray is performed and shows bilateral hilar lymphadenopathy. An abdominal ultrasound shows splenomegaly, but no hepatomegaly. Using the Ann Arbor staging system, which of the following stages best describes this patient's lymphoma?

A. Stage II
B. Stage IIb
C. Stage III
D. Stage IIIb
E. Stage IV

12. A patient presents to hospital severely unwell. She has an extensive purpuric rash. Her blood tests show the following:

Haemoglobin:	86 g/L
Platelet count:	26×10^9/L
Prothrombin time (PT):	25 seconds
Activated partial thromboplastin time (APTT):	76 seconds
D-dimer:	5463 ng/ml
Fibrinogen:	0.3 g/L

Which of the following would you expect to see on this patient's blood film?

A. Auer rods
B. Spherocytes
C. Schistocytes
D. Bite cells
E. Hienz bodies

13. A patient with a background of systemic lupus erythematosus (SLE) presents to her doctor feeling tired. A full blood count was ordered and showed the following:

Haemoglobin: 66 g/L
Mean corpusclar volume (MCV):   104 fL
White cell count: 7.3×10^9/L
Platelet count: 78×10^9/L

Which of the following tests would confirm the underlying cause of this patient's anaemia?

A. Warm direct Coombs test
B. Cold direct Coombs test
C. Indirect Coombs test
D. Bone marrow biopsy
E. Haemoglobin electrophoresis

14. A 76-year-old woman presents to her doctor with lethargy and fatigue. On examination she is found to have enlarged non-tender cervical lymph nodes, and hepatosplenomegaly. Some investigations are ordered and a blood film shows smear cells. She is subsequently referred to a haematologist. During this period she becomes increasingly unwell, her lymph nodes increase in size and she begins to lose weight rapidly. Which of the following best describes the cause of her worsening symptoms?

A. Hodgkin's lymphoma
B. Blast transformation
C. Waldenstrom's macroglobulinaemia
D. Richter's syndrome
E. Reiter's syndrome

15. A 6-year-old boy with cystic fibrosis presents with increased bruising on his arms and legs. His mum is concerned because last week he had a graze on his knee and it took 20 minutes to stop bleeding. His clotting studies are below:

Prothrombin time (PT): 25 seconds
Activated partial thromboplastin time (APTT): 76 seconds

Which of the following should be used to treat this patient?

A. Desmopressin
B. Prednisolone
C. Fresh frozen plasma
D. Prothrombin complex concentrate
E. Vitamin K

16. A 60-year-old woman presents to her general practitioner (GP) and is concerned that she is feeling more tired than usual. On examination the GP notices conjunctival pallor, gum hypertrophy and a loss of sensation in her hands and feet. On questioning she reported the occasional tingling in her feet. Her blood tests and blood film show a megaloblastic anaemia. Which of the following may explain the cause of this patient's anaemia?

A. Phenytoin
B. Methotrexate
C. Acute myeloid leukaemia
D. Crohn's disease
E. Pernicious anaemia

17. Which of the following is not consistent with iron deficiency anaemia?

A. Angular stomatitis
B. Atrophic glossitis
C. Raised platelets
D. Dysphagia
E. Leukonychia

18. A patient recently diagnosed with coeliac disease is started on ferrous sulphate and folic acid supplements to treat an underlying anaemia. Following two weeks of treatment a blood film is performed. Which of the following should be expected as a result of the new drugs that have been started?

A. Howell-Jolly bodies
B. Polychromasia
C. Poikilocytosis
D. Anisocytosis
E. Target cells

19. A 23-year-old boy with severe Crohn's disease develops anaemia. He is currently feeling tired but has not reported any dyspnea, chest pain or palpitations. His blood test results are below:

Haemoglobin:	75 g/L
Mean corpusclar volume (MCV):	69 fL
Serum vitamin B12:	567 ng/ml
Serum folate:	15 ng/ml
Serum iron:	32 µg/dl
Serum ferritin:	110 µg/L
Transferrin saturation:	7%

Which of the following should be used to treat this patient's anaemia?

A. Ferrous sulphate
B. Intravenous iron dextran
C. Intramuscular hydroxocobalamin
D. Oral vitamin B12
E. Blood transfusion

20. A 22-year-old male with a presents to hospital with a fever and feeling generally unwell. On examination he has a palpable spleen and cervical lymphadenopathy. His initial blood tests show a normocytic anaemia with a haemoglobin of 64 g/L and a reticulocyte count of 7%. Which of the following is the most likely cause of this patient's anaemia?

A. Epstein-Barr virus (EBV) infection
B. Parvovirus B19 infection
C. Chronic lymphocytic leukaemia
D. Myelodysplastic syndrome
E. Splenic sequestration crisis

21. A 22-year-old male student is being treated for large B-cell lymphoma. He has just started his treatment with cyclophosphamide, hydroxydaunorubicin, vincristine (oncovin) and prednisolone (CHOP regime). He has remains in hospital for 24 hours for observation. His observations remain stable and his blood tests are also normal except for a mild neutrophilia. Which of the following is the most likely cause of his raised neutrophils?

A. Bone marrow invasion by the lymphoma
B. Chronic myeloid leukaemia
C. Infection following chemotherapy
D. Side effect of the CHOP regime
E. Hypersplenism

22. A 55-year-old male was admitted for urgent neurosurgery to treat a subarachnoid haemorrhage. Five days post-operation he develops pain and swelling in his left leg. A venous doppler confirms the presence of a deep vein thrombosis (DVT). Which of the following treatment regimes is most appropriate?

A. Insertion of an inferior vena cava (IVC) filter
B. Dabigatran for 3 months
C. Dalteparin for 5 days followed by warfarin for 3 months
D. Dalteparin for 3 months
E. Initiate unfractionated heparin at treatment dose

23. A 45-year-old man is diagnosed with stable angina and started on long-term low dose aspirin. Since starting he has felt lethargic and a yellow tinge can be seen in his sclera. His blood tests show a normocytic anaemia, raised reticulocyte count and a raised unconjugated bilirubin, with otherwise normal liver function tests. On taking a detailed family history he reveals his grandfather also reacted in a similar fashion when prescribed some antibiotics. Which of the following is the most likely underlying diagnosis?

A. Glucose-6-phosphate dehydrogenase (G6PD) deficiency
B. Hereditary spherocytosis
C. Sickle cell disease
D. Folate deficiency
E. Warm haemolytic anaemia

24. A 30-year-old Turkish lady presents to her doctor complaining of tiredness and breathlessness on exertion. Her blood tests show the following:

Haemoglobin:	60 g/L
Mean corpusclar volume (MCV):	76 fL
Blood film:	target cells and pencil cells

Which of the following is the most likely diagnosis?

A. Beta thalassaemia trait
B. Sickle cell trait
C. Glucose-6-phosphate dehydrogenase (G6PD) deficiency
D. Iron deficiency anaemia (IDA)
E. Anaemia of chronic disease

25. A 67-year-old gentleman is being investigated for anaemia. On examination he doesn't have any palpable lymphadenopathy or any hepatosplenomegaly, but he does have some lumbar spine tenderness. His initial blood tests show a normocytic anaemia and chronic kidney disease (CKD) stage 4. Which of the following is the most likely diagnosis?

A. Diffuse large B cell lymphoma
B. Chronic myeloid leukaemia
C. Chronic lymphocytic leukaemia
D. Multiple myeloma
E. Myelofibrosis

26. A 10-year-old child with a history of sickle cell disease presents to hospital generally feeling unwell. On examination she is found to have an erythematous rash on both her cheeks and a high respiratory rate. Her blood tests show a normocytic anaemia, with no reticulocytes present. Which of the following is most likely to have caused her most recent symptoms?

A. Acute chest syndrome
B. Sequestration crisis
C. Parvovirus B19 infection
D. Rubella infection
E. Systemic lupus erythematosus (SLE)

27. A 22-year-old male presents to hospital with a fever 7 days after his first cycle of chemotherapy to treat Hodgkin's lymphoma. Which of the following is the most appropriate first step in this patient's management?

A. Intravenous 0.9% saline and allopurinol
B. Intravenous piperacillin/tazobactam and gentamicin
C. Intravenous trimethoprim with sulfamethoxazole
D. Intravenous ceftriaxone and dexamethasone
E. Granulocyte-colony stimulating factor (G-CSF)

28. A three-year-old African child presents to his doctor with fevers, night sweats and weight loss. On examination he is found to have a swollen jaw. His only significant past medical history is a positive monospot test, which was performed one year ago. What is the most likely diagnosis?

A. Acute lymphoblastic leukaemia (ALL)
B. Burkitt lymphoma
C. Hodgkin's lymphoma
D. Osteomyelitis
E. Avascular necrosis of the jaw

29. A 35-year-old man is given a blood transfusion. Shortly following the start of the blood transfusion he develops a fever, hypotension and blood begins to ooze from the cannula site. Which of the following should be given?

A. Intravenous dexamethasone
B. Intravenous 0.9% saline
C. Intravenous broad-spectrum antibiotics
D. Intravenous chlorpheniramine
E. Intravenous cryoprecipitate

30. A 70-year-old male presents with recurrent infections, easy bruising, weight loss and lethargy. Whilst in hospital he develops disseminated intravascular coagulation. He is subsequently diagnosed with acute promyelocytic leukaemia. Which of the following drugs is most likely to be prescribed?

A. All-trans retinoic acid
B. Imatinib
C. Prednisolone
D. Vitamin K
E. Protamine sulphate

Haematology Answers

1. A
Ferrous sulphate

This woman is describing symptoms of hypothyroidism. If ferrous sulphate is taken within two hours of levothyroxine then the absorption of levothyroxine is reduced, resulting in hypothyroidism. Ferrous sulphate can be given to treat iron deficiency anaemia for example in patients who don't have sufficient dietary intake or who have menorrhagia. None of the other medications listed would affect the absorption of levothyroxine.

Folic acid supplementation would be given in patients who have folate deficiency.

Oral vitamin B12 would be used in patients who have developed vitamin B12 deficiency due to insufficient dietary intake, such as in patents who have a vegan diet.

Intramusclar hydroxocobalamin is given to patients who are vitamin B12 deficient due to being unable to absorb vitamin B12 in the gut such as in pernicious anaemia or Crohn's disease.

Erythropoietin is given to patients who have chronic kidney disease and therefore don't produce enough of the hormone naturally.

2. D
Urea and creatinine

Rivaroxaban is a direct oral anticoagulant (DOAC) that inhibits factor Xa. The DOACs do not require regular monitoring of clotting, but because they are all excreted by the kidneys, patients should have at least annual monitoring of their renal function.

International normalised ratio (INR) is used to monitor warfarin and to guide the dose of warfarin that should be prescribed.

Activated partial thromboplastin time (APTT) ratio is used to monitor heparin infusions. Often it is measured every four hours while a heparin infusion is running and the value is used to adjust the dose of heparin.

Full blood count would be monitored in patients taking medications that can cause myelosuppression such as methotrexate and azathioprine.

Total cholesterol would be monitored in patients taking statins.

3. B
Acquired haemophilia

This patient's plasma has been mixed with normal plasma in a 50/50 ratio. If this causes the APTT to decrease by more than 4 seconds it would mean there is a deficiency in one of the clotting factors. However, if it doesn't cause a decrease in the APTT, it means there is something inhibiting the pathway, such as acquired haemophilia or antiphospholipid syndrome. Acquired haemophilia is an autoimmune condition occurring in both males and females, where there is production of anti-factor VIII antibodies. It causes a raised APTT and factor VIII activity <50%. It is treated with corticosteroids.

Antiphospholipid syndrome is procoagulant and patients are at risk of both arterial and venous thrombosis, therefore it wouldn't cause bleeding. However it is associated with thrombocytopenia and also a raised APTT. The raised APTT is due to the presence of lupus anticoagulant. In-vitro this acts to raise the APTT, however in-vivo it is a procoagulant.

Von Willebrand's disease is a genetic condition that causes a lack of von Willebrand factor (vWF). There are three types: type 1 is due to reduced levels of vWF, and type 2 is due to abnormal vWF. Both of which are autosomal dominant. Type 3 causes undetectable levels of vWF and is autosomal recessive. Blood tests show a slightly raised APTT, increased bleeding time, reduced factor VIII and reduced vWF. The APTT would improve on mixing the plasma with normal plasma.

Vitamin K deficiency would lead to a lack of factors II, VII, IX and X, which are all vitamin K dependent. This mainly affects the extrinsic pathway leading to a raised international normalised ratio (INR) and raised prothrombin time.

4. D
Reduced neutrophil alkaline phosphatase

Neutrophil alkaline phosphatase is present in high concentrations in normal neutrophils, but it is reduced or absent in malignant neutrophils. Therefore in chronic myeloid leukaemia it is reduced. This test is rarely used now because it is easy to test for the Philadelphia chromosome. This is a formed due to a t(9;22) translocation, which forms the BCR-ABL gene. This has tyrosine kinase activity and therefore imatinib (a tyrosine kinase inhibitor) can be used to treat chronic myeloid leukaemia. The neutrophil alkaline phosphatase can be used to differentiate chronic myeloid leukaemia from polycythaemia ruba vera, where it would be raised.

JAK2 mutations can be found in the other myeloproliferative disorders such as polycythaemia rubra vera and essential thrombocythaemia.

A right shift is where there are hypermature white cells seen on the peripheral blood film, and this occurs in vitamin B12 deficiency, liver disease and uraemia. These cells have hyper-segmented nuclei (>5 lobes per nuclei).

Cervical lymphadenopathy is more likely in chronic lymphocytic leukaemia (CLL). A lymphocytosis describes raised lymphocytes, which is also more likely in CLL. Patients with CML have increased levels of white blood cells from the myeloid cell lines such as neutrophils.

5. A
Idiopathic thrombocytopenic purpura (ITP)

This patient has developed idiopathic thrombocytopenic purpura (ITP), which presents with easy bruising, a purpuric rash, bleeding from the gums or nose, and menorrhagia. In ITP antibodies are produced which bind to the platelets and lead to platelet destruction in the spleen. It can occur following a recent viral infection such as Epstein-Barr virus (EBV), cytomegalovirus (CMV), human immunodeficiency virus (HIV) or in autoimmune diseases such as in systemic lupus erythematosus (SLE), but often a cause isn't found.

Thrombotic thrombocytopenic purpura (TTP) presents with fever, fluctuating central nervous system signs, microangiopathic haemolytic anaemia (MAHA) and acute kidney injury. TTP is caused by a deficiency in ADAMTS13, an enzyme responsible for cleaving von Willebrand factor (vWF) into smaller units. The circulating large multimers of vWF increase platelet binding to the endothelium of blood vessels causing the formation of multiple thrombi and also using up the circulating platelets and leaving the patient at risk of bleeding.

Meningococcal septicaemia can cause low platelets by disseminated intravascular coagulation (DIC), but these patients would present very unwell, with a high fever and septic shock.

Haemophilia A is an X-linked deficiency in factor VIII, and wouldn't cause a low platelet count.

Liver cirrhosis can lead to a low platelet count through portal hypertension causing hypersplenism, but would also present with other signs of liver disease such as jaundice and ascites.

6. D
Danaparoid or lepirudin

This patient has developed heparin-induced thrombocytopenia. This occurs 5–10 days after being given heparin (or less commonly low molecular weight heparin), and results in antibodies being produced against the platelets. It causes the patient to become prothrombotic, thrombocytopenic (often over a 50% reduction in platelet number), and skin reactions can also occur. Treatment is to stop the heparin and give danaparoid (a factor Xa inhibitor) or lepirudin (a direct thrombin inhibitor).

Protamine sulphate can be used to reverse the anticoagulant actions of heparin.

7. D
Hypokalaemia

Heparin can cause hyperkalaemia because it inhibits the activity of aldosterone. It can cause thrombocytopenia due to heparin-induced thrombocytopenia; haemorrhage due to reducing the activity of the clotting cascade, urticaria due to hypersenstitivity and it can also cause osteoporosis.

8. B
Raised HbA$_2$

This patient has thalassaemia minor/trait, which is the carrier state of the mutant β-globin chain. It presents with a microcytic anaemia. The anaemia is mild (haemoglobin > 90 g/L) and asymptomatic. It is diagnosed by electrophoresis showing a raised HbA$_2$. There is also a slight rise in HbF. In thalassaemia major there is a raised HbF, variable HbA$_2$, and HbA is absent. The blood film would show anisocytosis, poikilocytosis and target cells.

Polychromasia is where the red blood cells are of different ages and thus they stain differently, such as in reticulocytosis caused by a haemolytic anaemia.

Pappenheimer bodies are abnormal basophilic granules of iron inside red blood cells, which are seen post-splenectomy. Other signs of hyposplenism on a blood film include target cells and Howell-Jolly bodies.

9. A
Erythromycin

This patient has developed ciclosporin toxicity and has presented with acute kidney injury as a result of nephrotoxicity, and a tremor. Other side effects include hypertension, oedema, hepatotoxicity, hyperkalaemia, seizures and an increased risk of lymphoma and skin cancer. Ciclosporin is metabolised by the P450 system, and therefore any P450 inhibitors can increase its plasma concentration: such as amioderone, verapamil, cimetidine, erythromycin and ketoconazole.

The other drugs listed all decrease the plasma concentration of ciclosporin. Griseofulvin, phenytoin and carbamazepine are all P450 inducers. Other P450 inducers include rifampicin, chronic alcohol use, phenobarbitone and sulphonylureas.

10. C
Leukoerythroblastic cells

This patient has developed myelofibrosis, which is hyperplasia of the megakaryocytes. It presents with B symptoms (fevers, weight loss and night sweats) and massive hepatosplenomegaly. It can follow on from other myeloproliferative disorders, such as essential thrombocythaemia. The blood film shows leukoerythroblastic cells, which are immature white cells and tear drop red blood cells.

Auer rods are found in acute myeloid leukaemia.

> Mirror cells are found in acute lymphocytic leukaemia.
>
> Rouleaux formation is where red blood cells stack upon each other and occurs in any condition causing a paraproteinaemia such as multiple myeloma, Waldenstrom's macroglobulinaemia, chronic lymphocytic leukaemia and lymphomas.
>
> Left shift is where immature neutrophils are sent out of the bone marrow, such as in infection, and they are released early before they have time to fully mature.

11. D
Stage IIIb

This patient has B symptoms (fevers, night sweats and weight loss). Stage 1 is where only one lymph node is affected; stage 2 is where two or more lymph nodes on the same side of the diaphragm are affected, stage 3 is where lymph nodes on either side of the diaphragm are affected (the spleen is regarded as a lymph node in this scoring system), and stage 4 is where there is extra-nodal involvement, such as the liver or bone.

This patent has bilateral hilar lymphadenopathy and splenomegaly, therefore lymph nodes on either side of the diaphragm are involved and along with the B symptoms this would be stage IIIb.

Other important differentials for bilateral hilar lymphadenopathy are tuberculosis and sarcoidosis; less common causes include extrinsic allergic alveolitis (which has more recently been renamed as hypersensitivity pneumonitis), and organic dust disease such as silicosis and berylliosis.

12. C
Schistocytes

This patient has disseminated intravascular coagulation (DIC). This presents with a purpuric rash and blood tests show a low platelet count, low fibrinogen, raised PT, APTT, bleeding time and D-dimer. This is because of the increased coagulation leading to the clotting factors being used up. Schistocytes are fragmented red blood cells, which are sliced by fibrin strands as they try to move past the thrombus, and these are found in any cause of microangiopathic haemolytic anaemia, such as DIC, haemolytic uraemia syndrome and thrombotic thrombocytopenic purpura.

Spherocytes are round red blood cells, found in hereditary spherocytosis and warm autoimmune haemolytic anaemia.

Bite cells and Hienz bodies are present in glucose-6-phosphate dehydrogenase (G6PD) deficiency. Heinz bodies describe the inclusions found in red blood cells, that occur as a result of free radicals causing haemoglobin to become denatured. Heinz bodies are removed by the spleen resulting in formation of bite cells and blister cells.

13. A
Warm direct Coombs test

This patient has developed a warm haemolytic anaemia as a result of SLE. Other causes of a warm haemolytic anaemia include chronic lymphocytic leukaemia, and drugs such as methyldopa, but most commonly it is idiopathic. The warm direct Coombs test is where a patient's red blood cells (RBCs) are washed, and then incubated with anti-human antibodies (Coombs reagent). Then if the RBCs agglutinate it means there were auto-antibodies stuck to the wall of the RBCs. If this occurs at a warm temperature it is warm direct Coombs test positive, and if it occurs at a cold temperature it is cold direct Coombs test positive. A cold direct Coombs test would identify cold haemolytic anaemias such as those caused by Epstein-Barr virus (EBV) and Mycoplasma pneumoniae.

Indirect Coombs test is used to determine a patient's blood type for a transfusion. A patient's serum is taken and the donor's blood is added to the serum, followed by the Coombs reagent. If there is a reaction it means that the patient's serum must contain antibodies against the donor's RBCs. Thus it can be used to determine a patient's blood type.

Bone marrow biopsy would be to look at the composition of the bone marrow such as in leukaemias.

Haemoglobin electrophoresis is used to look at the composition of the haemoglobin chain and is used to diagnose thalaessaemia and sickle cell disease.

14. D
Richter's syndrome

This patient has got an underlying diagnosis of chronic lymphocytic leukaemia (CLL). This is evident because of the signs found on examination and the smear cells on the blood film. These are fragile lymphocytes that smear on the peripheral blood film. Most people with CLL either die as a result of infection, or because of transformation to an aggressive lymphoma, which is known as Richter's syndrome. This is evident here because of the rapid deterioration and increasing size of lymph nodes, making this the most likely diagnosis.

A blast transformation occurs in chronic myeloid leukaemia (CML) and is where the CML begins to act like an acute leukaemia and release blast cells into the blood. CML has three main phases: a chronic phases lasting months or years which is either asymptomatic or has few symptoms, an accelerated phase where there is increasing symptoms, increasing spleen size and rising white cell counts, and last is the blast transformation.

Waldenstrom's macroglobulinaemia is a malignant proliferation of B-cells resulting in an IgM paraprotein. This presents similarly to multiple myeloma with symptoms of hyperviscocity, but is more likely to cause organomegaly and less likely to cause hypercalcaemia.

15. E
Vitamin K

Cystic fibrosis is an autosomal recessive condition caused by a mutation in the cystic fibrosis transmembrane conductance regulator, which codes for a chloride channel. This can cause increased mucus production in the lungs leading to recurrent infections and bronchiectasis. It also causes pancreatic insufficiency, which can result in reduced enzyme production and fat soluble vitamin deficiencies. As a result this patient has developed a vitamin K deficiency. This is evident in the prolonged prothrombin time.

Desmopressin could be used as part of the treatment for haemophilia A, it is a vasopressin analogue which acts to increase release for factor VIII from the vascular endothelium.

Fresh frozen plasma is used to replace clotting factors in patients that are deficient.

Prothrombin complex concentrate contains the vitamin K dependent clotting factors II, VII, IX and X, as well as protein C and S. It can be used to rapidly reverse warfarin.

16. A
Phenytoin

Phenytoin is an anti-epileptic drug and can cause a folate deficiency, which can lead to a megaloblastic anaemia. Its other side effects include gum hypertrophy, coarse facial features, hirsutism, peripheral neuropathy (loss of sensation) and cerebellar atrophy (ataxia, dysdiadochokinesia, intention tremor, nystagmus, staccato or slurred speech)

A megaloblastic anaemia is due to either a folate or vitamin B12 deficiency. A megaloblast is a cell where the nuclear maturation is delayed compared to the cytoplasm. This occurs because both vitamin B12 and folate are required for DNA synthesis. It causes a macrocytosis and hyper-segmented neutrophils on the peripheral blood film.

Methotrexate can also cause a folate deficiency, and its side effects include teratogenicity, oral ulceration, bone marrow suppression, pulmonary and liver fibrosis.

Acute myeloid leukaemia can cause gum hypertrophy but it causes a normocytic normochromic anaemia. It is also more likely to present with bleeding, recurrent infections, and B-symptoms.

Crohn's disease can cause both vitamin B12 and folate deficiencies but doesn't cause gum hypertrophy. It would present with abdominal pain, bloody diarrhoea, oral ulceration and fistulae formation.

Pernicious anaemia is another cause of vitamin B12 deficiency. It is an autoimmune condition where auto-antibodies are produced against the intrinsic factor, which is required for vitamin B12 absorption. This would present with symptoms of anaemia and patients often have a background of other autoimmune diseases.

Causes of gum hypertrophy include scurvy, pregnancy, acute myeloid leukaemia, phenytoin, nifedipine, tacrolimus and ciclosporin.

17. E
Leukonychia

Leukonychia is caused by hypoalbuminaemia, and is the white discoloration of the nails.

Dysphagia occurs as part of Plummer-Vinson syndrome, which is the triad of dysphagia, oesophageal post cricoids webs and iron deficiency anaemia (IDA). Plummer-Vinson syndrome is associated with an increased risk of oesophageal cancer.

Angular stomatitis can occur in IDA and in both vitamin B2 and vitamin B12 deficiency.

Atrophic glossitis occurs in IDA, whereas a red beefy tongue may be seen in vitamin B12 deficiency.

Raised platelets can occur in IDA, chronic inflammatory conditions, infection, bleeding, malignancy and essential thrombocythaemia.

18. B
Polychromasia

Polychromasia is the formation of red blood cells of different ages. The red blood cells stain different colours on the blood film, with the younger cells staining bluer. This can occur in haematinic replacement (iron, vitamin B12 and folate), haemolysis, bleeding and bone marrow infiltration. A reticulocytosis is also likely to be present.

Howell-Jolly bodies are found in hyposplenism.

Target cells are present in iron deficiency anaemia (IDA), thalassaemia and hyposplenism.

Poikilocytosis is red blood cells of different shapes, found in IDA, thalassaemia and myelofibrosis.

Anisocytosis is red blood cells of different sizes, found in IDA, thalassaemia and megaloblastic anaemia.

19. B
Intravenous iron dextran

This patient has a microcytic anaemia. The most common cause of this is iron deficiency. This is confirmed by the low serum iron and low transferrin saturation, and is likely to be due to malabsorption as a result of inflammatory bowel disease. The ferritin should be low; however it is raised due to the ongoing inflammation, therefore overall it is within the normal range. Normally oral ferrous supplements are used; however due to the small intestine being unable to absorb iron, the only way this person can be given iron is intravenously.

A blood transfusion is not required because the anaemia is not very severe. Normally it would be considered in someone who is symptomatic or with a haemoglobin of less that 70 g/L.

Intramuscular hydroxocobalamin is given to patients who are vitamin B12 deficient but can't absorb oral supplements, such as in pernicious anaemia, or if Crohn's disease has caused vitamin B12 deficiency.

Oral vitamin B12 is often given to vegans, who don't have any underlying digestive pathology. They are able to absorb oral vitamin B12, but are deficient because of their diet.

20. C
Epstein-Barr virus (EBV) infection

This patient has developed a haemolytic anaemia as a result of an EBV infection. In haemolysis the blood tests would show a raised reticulocyte count, as the bone marrow would be releasing immature red cells to try and compensate for the rapid decrease in haemoglobin. This patient would also have a raised unconjugated bilirubin, raised serum lactate dehydrogenase (LDH) and a reduced serum haptoglobin.

Chronic lymphocytic leukaemia can also cause a haemolytic anaemia, however it presents in elderly patients and therefore is not the underlying diagnosis in this case.

A parvovirus B19 infection can cause an aplastic crisis is where the bone marrow is unable to produce any new blood cells. Patients with pre-existing conditions such as sickle cell disease, require a high rate of erythropoiesis to maintain their haemoglobin level, due to the reduced lifespan of their red blood cells. Therefore they are at a higher risk of developing an aplastic crisis. It presents with anaemia and a reduced reticulocyte count.

A splenic sequestration crisis can occur in young children with sickle cell disease, and is due to the sequestration of red cells in the spleen causing splenic infarction. By adulthood the spleen will have auto-infarcted and therefore splenic sequestration will no longer occur.

Myelodysplastic syndrome occurs in elderly patients and is due to the dysfunction of the bone marrow. It can lead to disruption of multiple cell lines causing a pancytopenia. Some cases develop into an acute myeloid leukaemia.

21. D
Side effect of the CHOP regime

This patient has been started on prednisolone as part of his chemotherapy regime. All corticosteroids act to cause detachment of neutrophils from the endothelial lining of the blood vessels. Neutrophils are normally present in the circulating blood or rolling along the endothelial lining of the vessels. When a blood sample is taken only the cells in the circulating blood are measured. Corticosteroids increase the number circulating as they cause the neutrophils to detach from the endothelial walls. Therefore the rise in number seen on a full blood count is not a true rise, just something that is seen in the blood test.

Chemotherapy can cause neutopenia due to bone marrow suppression, but this is most common 7 days after therapy.

Infections can occur following chemotherapy, due to neutropenia. This is most likely 7 days after chemotherapy and would show low neutrophils on the blood count. Also the patient would have a fever.

Bone marrow invasion by the lymphoma would also cause low neutrophils, and is likely to affect the other cell lines causing anaemia and low platelets.

Hypersplenism would also cause a low neutrophil count due to cells pooling in the spleen and being destroyed by the reticuloendothelial system. This can occur in lymphomas, leukaemias, myeloproliferative disorders, and also autoimmune conditions such as Felty's syndrome, systemic lupus erythematosus (SLE) and autoimmune haemolysis. Infections that cause it include malaria and Epstein–Barr virus (EBV). Hypersplenism can also be due to increased splenic blood flow such as in liver cirrhosis.

Chronic myeloid leukaemia is a cause of neutrophilia, as it is a malignancy of the myeloid precursor cells. However it occurs in older patients. Also the neutrophils would be markedly raised, and immature cells would have also been reported. This is a separate condition to lymphoma, and extremely unlikely in a patient this young.

22. A
Insertion of an inferior vena cava (IVC) filter

This patient has recently had an intracranial bleed and therefore all forms of anticoagulation are contraindicated. An IVC filter would act to prevent the DVT from embolising to the lungs. All other options involve anticoagulation and therefore aren't appropriate.

23. A
Glucose-6-phosphate dehydrogenase (G6PD) deficiency

This patient has developed a haemolytic anaemia. This is evident because of the normocytic anaemia, raised reticulocyte count and jaundice caused by raised unconjugated bilirubin. If the reticulocyte count is high enough a haemolytic anaemia can cause a macrocytic anaemia. G6PD deficiency is an X-linked condition that leads to reduced glutathione production in the red blood cells. This can cause a crisis due to oxidative damage. The damage leads to production of Heinz bodies and in turn bite and blister cells. It can be precipitated by drugs such as aspirin, sulphonamides, dapsone and primaquine, and also by illness and ingestion of fava beans. It is likely his grandfather was prescribed a sulphonamide and had a similar reaction.

Hereditary spherocytosis is autosomal dominant and causes a haemolytic anaemia and splenomegaly. This is less likely because aspirin caused this particular episode.

Sickle cell anaemia is an autosomal recessive condition caused by a genetic mutation in the make up of the beta haemoglobin chains. This leads to sequestration of the haemoglobin and a crisis that can be precipitated by hypoxia, acidosis, dehydration and infection.

Autoimmune antibodies being produced against the red blood cells cause a warm haemolytic anaemia. This is less likely due to this case having a clear family history. Also aspirin doesn't cause an autoimmune haemolytic anaemia. Drugs responsible include methyldopa, ribavirin and penicillins.

24. D
Iron deficiency anaemia (IDA)

This patent has a microcytic anaemia due to the MCV < 80 fL. Of the causes of anaemia listed only three would cause a microcytic anaemia: beta thalassaemia trait, IDA and anaemia of chronic disease. Beta thalassaemia trait causes a very low MCV, relative to the severity of the anaemia. Often the anaemia is mild and asymptomatic (haemoglobin > 90 g/L) but the MCV is very low (MCV < 75 fL). Therefore this is unlikely. Anaemia of chronic disease is also unlikely because there is no history of any other medical conditions. IDA is therefore most likely, and it is also a cause of target cells and pencil cells on the blood film. Other causes of target cells include hyposplenism, liver failure and thalassaemia. Pencil cells can also be seen in thalassaemia.

Sickle cell disease is an autosomal recessive condition. If a patient is a carrier they are known as having sickle cell trait, and are often asymptomatic. Also this would cause a normocytic anaemia and therefore it is unlikely. Also sickle cells would be seen on the blood film.

G6PD deficiency is an X-linked recessive condition and therefore only occurs in males. It causes a haemolytic anaemia and therefore would either cause a normocytic or macrocytic anaemia due to reticulocytosis.

25. D
Multiple myeloma

Multiple myeloma should be considered in any elderly patient with anaemia and back pain. It is due to the uncontrolled clonal proliferation of plasma cells and is characterised by the frequent development of osteolytic bone lesions (often in the spine causing back pain), renal failure, anaemia, hypercalcaemia and amyloidosis.

Diffuse large B-cell lymphoma and chronic lymphocytic leukaemia would both present with lymphadenopathy, due to the underlying proliferation of lymphocytes.

Chronic myeloid leukaemia is most commonly caused by the translocation of the 9th and 22nd chromosomes leading to formation of the Philadelphia chromosome. It leads to formation of the BCR-ABL gene and over production of myeloid cells in the bone marrow. These patients develop massive hepatosplenomegaly and very high white cell counts.

Myelofibrosis is a bone marrow disorder where production of cytokines leads to abnormal megakaryocytes and replacement of normal haematopoietic bone marrow tissue with connective tissue. Myeloproliferative conditions such as polycythaemia rubra vera, and essential thrombocythaemia that occur secondary to the JAK2 mutation can develop into myelofibrosis. It leads to bone marrow failure and pancytopenia, and presents with hepatosplenomegaly, fevers, weight loss and night sweats.

26. C
Parvovirus B19 infection

Parvovirus B19 causes 'slapped cheek syndrome', and presents with a malar rash, fever and lethargy. It is most often a mild infection, but in patients with sickle cell it can cause an aplastic anaemia. This presents with a normocytic anaemia and a lack of reticulocytes. This patient may require a blood transfusion. She has a high respiratory rate due to the anaemia, suggesting it is severe.

Acute chest syndrome occurs in sickle cell disease due to pulmonary infiltrates occurring as a result of a vaso-occlusive crisis affecting the pulmonary vasculature. It can occur as a result of atypical infections such as Chlamydia pneumoniae, Mycoplasma pneumoniae or respiratory viruses, or due to a fat embolism. It presents with chest pain, fever, tachypnoea, cough and wheeze.

Sequestration crisis is where there is a vaso-occulsive crisis in the spleen. There is pooling of the blood in the spleen causing splenomegaly, anaemia and shock. This occurs in young patients, as once patients get older splenic atrophy is likely to have occurred.

Rubella is an RNA virus, which causes a fever, macular rash and suboccipital lymphadenopathy. However it wouldn't cause an aplastic anaemia.

Systemic lupus erythematosus (SLE) is a multisystem autoimmune condition. Its features include malar rash, photosensitive rash, alopecia, oral ulceration, polyarthritis, pleurisy, pericarditis, and glomerulonephritis. It can also cause a warm autoimmune haemolytic anaemia. However a haemolytic anaemia would cause a raised reticulocyte count.

27. B
Intravenous piperacillin/tazobactam and gentamicin

This patient has suspected neutropenic sepsis. Any patient that presents with a fever following chemotherapy should be treated as having neutropenic sepsis until proven otherwise. It is most common between 5–10 days after chemotherapy. The mainstay of treatment is broad spectrum antibiotics (such as piperacillin/tazobactam and gentamicin). Treatment also includes barrier nursing and trying to isolate the cause of infection by taking blood cultures prior to the first dose of antibiotics. G-CSF can be given to stimulate neutrophil production but would only be considered once antibiotics have been administered.

Ceftriaxone and dexamethasone would be used to treat meningitis. Dexamethasone is given to prevent deafness.

Trimethoprim with sulfamethoxazole is also known as co-trimoxazole and may be given if a Pneumocystis jirovecii infection is suspected.

Intravenous 0.9% saline and allopurinol would be used to treat tumour lysis syndrome. This occurs following chemotherapy due to the rapid destruction of cells. It causes raised serum potassium, raised serum urate, raised serum phosphate and low serum calcium. It can lead to acute kidney injury so fluids are extremely important.

28. B
Burkitt lypmphoma

Burkitt's lymphoma is a rapidly progressive, high grade non-Hodgkin's lymphoma which mainly affects children in Africa. It is associated with a previous Epstein–Barr virus (EBV) infection (tested for by a mono-spot test). It classically causes swelling of the jaw.

Hodgkin's lymphoma is more common in slightly older patients, and also in elderly adults due to its two peaks of incidence. It presents with painless rubbery lymph nodes and B-symptoms.

Acute lymphoblastic leukaemia (ALL) is most common in young children and can also cause lymphadenopathy, organomegaly, bilateral parotid swelling, orchidomegaly and if it invades the central nervous system it can cause cranial nerve palsies and meningism.

Osteomyelitis is an infection of the bone. Patients with diabetes mellitus, immunosuppression and sickle cell disease are more prone to developing it, but there are no predisposing factors to suggest this.

Avascular necrosis of the jaw is death of the bone as a result of a lack of blood supply. Causes include sickle cell disease, steroids, alcohol, radiotherapy and arterial embolism. Avascular necrosis of the jaw is also a specific side effect of bisphosphonates.

29. B
Intravenous 0.9% saline

This patient has developed a haemolytic transfusion reaction. This has occurred due to a cross reaction between the patient's plasma antibodies and the ABO antigens present on the donors red blood cells. It presents with a fever, hypotension, tachycardia, flushing, abdominal and chest pain, oozing from the venipuncture site and it can progress to disseminated intravascular coagulation (DIC). Treatment is to stop the transfusion immediately and start intravenous 0.9% saline.

Intravenous dexamethasone is a strong steroid used to reduce inflammation and oedema. It doesn't have a role in treating acute haemolytic reactions.

Intravenous broad-spectrum antibiotics would be given if an infection were suspected. This is most common in platelet transfusions, because platelets are stored at 22 degrees Celsius and are prone to being contaminated.

Intravenous chlorpheniramine is an antihistamine used to treat allergic and anaphylactic reactions. This occurs in patents that lack IgA, producing anti-IgA antibodies against the donors IgA. Allergies cause urticaria and puritis and can progress to anaphylaxis, which presents with bronchospasm, cyanosis, hypotension and angioedema.

Intravenous cryoprecipitate is a combination of fibrinogen, factor VIII and von Willebrand's factor. It is used to treat DIC, because it is a good source of fibrinogen, which becomes depleted in DIC.

30. A
All-trans retinoic acid

Acute promyelocytic leukaemia (APML) is the M3 subtype of acute myeloid leukaemia (AML) and is caused by a t(15; 17) translocation, which creates the retinoic acid receptor-alpha (*RARA*), promyelocytic leukaemia gene (PML). It presents with similar symptoms to AML but these patients are also prone to developing disseminated intravascular coagulation (DIC). All-trans retinoid acid is a form of vitamin A that binds to the RARA receptor and prevents the mutated gene from having an effect. This is combined with other chemotherapy agents to induce remission. APML can be differentiated from other forms of AML by its response to all-trans retinoid acid.

Imatinib is a tyrosine kinase inhibitor used to treat chronic myeloid leukaemia, caused by the Philadelphia chromosome.

Prednisolone is a steroid used in immunosuppression, and to treat non-Hodgkin's lymphoma as part of the CHOP regime.

Vitamin K can be given in vitamin K deficiency and also to reverse warfarin.

Protamine sulphate is a drug given to reverse unfractionated heparin.

Infectious Diseases Questions

1. A 19-year-old student presents to hospital a week after returning from a gap year in South America with dysphagia. He is unable to swallow solids or liquids, and a barium swallow shows a bird beak appearance. On examination his abdomen was found to be grossly distended and tender. Abdominal X-ray showed dilated loops of large bowel. Which organism has this patient been infected with whilst travelling?

A. Trypanosoma gambiense
B. Trypanosoma cruzi
C. Leishmania braziliensis
D. Clostridium tetani
E. Polio virus

2. A 28-year-old woman presents to her doctor following her honeymoon in the Seychelles. She describes having abdominal pain and diarrhoea for the last few weeks, and she has also developed a cough and a wheeze recently. On examination the doctor finds a rash, which the patient then states has moved location since it first began a few weeks ago. Her blood tests show an eosinophilia. Which drug should she be prescribed to treat the underlying infection?

A. Metronidazole
B. Praziquantel
C. Amphotericin B
D. Ivermectin
E. Ceftriaxone

3. A 45-year-old male presents to his doctor following a holiday in Tanzania with frequency, haematuria and haematospermia. Prior to this he felt generally unwell for two weeks. Whilst away on holiday he went on various day trips and swam in Lake Malawi. What drug should the doctor prescribe to treat the underlying infection?

A. Trimethorprim
B. Azithromycin
C. Praziquantel
D. Cephalexin
E. Fluconazole

4. A woman presents to hospital following a recent trip to India. She has a fever, abdominal pain and green diarrhea. She also has a dry cough and a sparse 'rose spots' across her chest. Blood cultures confirm a diagnosis of Salmonella typhi. Which of the following medications should be used to treat the underlying infection?

A. Amoxicillin
B. Ceftriaxone
C. Metronidazole
D. Clarithromycin
E. Ivermectin

5. A 34-year-old woman presents to hospital with severe abdominal pain two days after a summer barbecue. She also described having bloody diarrhoea. A stool sample is taken and microscopy shows multiple gram-negative spiral rods. What is the organism most likely to be causing her symptoms?

A. Bacillus cereus
B. Staphylococcus aureus
C. Escherichia coli
D. Campylobacter jejuni
E. Salmonella enteritidis

6. A 21-year-old student returned from a holiday in Russia. Two weeks later he began to have diarrhoea. This continued for two weeks until he decided to see his doctor. By this point he had lost a significant amount of weight. He described his stool as large, bulky and difficult to flush, but there was no blood present. He also stated the two friends he travelled with were also experiencing similar symptoms. Which of the following drugs should he be prescribed?

A. Tinidazole
B. Fluconazole
C. Co-trimoxazole
D. Ciprofloxacin
E. Erythromycin

7. A 54-year-old man with severe human immunodeficiency virus (HIV) is brought into doctor. He has become increasingly confused over the past few weeks, and has spent a lot of time in his room with his curtains drawn. Two days ago he began vomiting. On examination he is found to have bilateral sixth cranial nerve palsies, but no neck stiffness. Blood tests reveal a CD4 count of 90 cells/μL and negative interferon gamma release assay (IGRA). A CT scan of his head showed signs of raised intracranial pressure, but no focal lesions. His lumbar puncture revealed a raised opening pressure of 45 mmHg. What is the organism most likely to be causing his symptoms?

A. Toxoplasma gondii
B. Cryptococcus neoformans
C. Mycobacterium tuberculosis
D. Cytomegalovirus
E. Herpes simplex virus

8. A 35-year-old mother takes her 5-year-old child to hospital. Her child is subsequently diagnosed with meningococcal meningitis. The mother is worried that she may have also contracted the infection. The doctor decides to prescribe her some prophylactic medication. Her only significant past medical history is that she is currently recovering from a hepatitis A infection and as a result is slightly jaundiced. Which drug should be prescribed as prophylaxis?

A. Ceftriaxone
B. Metronidazole
C. Clarithromycin
D. Ciprofloxacin
E. Rifampicin

9. An alcoholic male is brought into hospital with a swinging fever and productive cough. He is producing foul smelling, green sputum. His chest X-ray shows a cavitating lesion in the left lower lobe, which contains a fluid level and his blood cultures have grown gram-negative rods. What is the organism most likely to be causing his symptoms?

A. Streptococcus pneumoniae
B. Staphylococcus aureus
C. Mycobacterium tuberculosis
D. Klebsiella pneumoniae
E. Pseudomonas aeruginosa

10. A 10-year-old child who was born immigrated to the United Kingdom recently and has never been vaccinated presents to hospital with a sore throat and a cough. On examination he has a fever, grey plaques on his tonsils and neck swelling from cervical lymphadenopathy. He doesn't have any rashes or joint pains. Which of the following is the most likely diagnosis?

A. Rheumatic fever
B. Measles
C. Rubella
D. Polio
E. Diphtheria

11. A 24-year-old student returns early from his travelling due to bloody diarrhoea that started a few weeks ago. He presents to hospital with a high swinging fever and night sweats. On examination the patient is found to have right upper quadrant pain, an an enlarged liver and jaundice. An ultrasound scan of his abdomen confirms the presence of a liver abscess. What is the most likely underlying pathogen?

A. Hepatitis A virus
B. Cytomegalovirus
C. Mycobacterium tuberculosis
D. Schistosoma mansoni
E. Entamoeba histolytica

12. An elderly lady presents with new onset confusion and a fever. On examination she was unable to move her head and also expressed discomfort when the doctor tried to examine her eyes with an ophthalmoscope. However there were no signs of papilledema. As part of her workup a lumber puncture is performed. The cerebrospinal fluid (CSF) results are below:

CSF microscopy and culture: Gram-positive bacilli
CSF white cell count: 250 cells/μL (90% lymphocytes)
CSF protein: 1 g/L
CSF glucose: 2.3 mmol/L

Which of the following regimes should be used to treat this patient?

A. Intravenous ceftriaxone
B. Intravenous ceftriaxone and dexamethasone with each dose of antibiotics
C. Intravenous ceftriaxone and ampicillin
D. Intravenous aciclovir
E. Rifampicin, isoniazid, pyrazinamide and ethambutol

13. A 35-year-old Nigerian immigrant, who recently moved to the United Kingdom, presents to his doctor with a penile ulcer. The ulcer is painful and tender. It has irregular jagged borders and a yellow granulomatous base. Which of the following is the underlying cause of this patient's ulcer?

A. Chlamydia trachomatis
B. Treponema pallidum
C. Klebsiella granulomatis
D. Haemophilus ducreyi
E. Herpes simplex

14. A 22-year-old male is brought into hospital following a collapse. His friend who witnessed his fall said he went pale and was unconscious for a minute before waking. He fully recovered within a couple of minutes. On full exposure a circular erythematous bull's-eye rash could be seen on his left arm. On questioning about the rash the patient stated that the rash was gradually getting larger. He also complained of widespread arthralgia, and was subsequently diagnosed with a Borrelia burgdorferi infection. What is the most likely cause of this patients collapse?

A. Vasovagal collapse
B. Hypoglycemia
C. Atrioventricular block
D. Aortic stenosis
E. Meningitis

15. A patient presents to his doctor with a hard painless genital ulcer, which had been present for a few weeks. He has more recently developed a maculopapular rash on his hands and feet. The doctor decided to treat him with procaine benzylpenicillin. Following the treatment the patient developed a high fever; tachycardia and he also noticed his genital ulcer becoming larger as a result. What is the most likely cause of his new symptoms?

A. Concurrent Epstein-Barr virus infection
B. Anaphylaxis
C. Contaminated medication causing sepsis
D. Jarish-Herxheimer reaction
E. Reiter's syndrome

16. A 56-year-old farmer is brought into hospital with a cough, chest pain and myalgia. On examination a subconjunctival haemorrhage could be seen in his left eye. Whilst in hospital he rapidly deteriorated. He became jaundiced and oliguric. Which of the following organisms is most likely to be causing this patient's symptoms?

A. Legionella pneumophila
B. Staphylococcus aureus
C. Bacillus anthracis
D. Leptospira interrogans
E. Epstein-Barr virus

17. A young male patient presents to hospital with a fever, sore throat, cough and pleuritic chest pain On examination he has a swollen and extremely tender neck, and is unable to open his mouth because it causes him too much pain. Therefore the doctor is unable to examine his throat. A computed tomography (CT) scan of his neck and chest is performed and shows a thrombus in the left internal jugular vein and a cavitating lesion in the right middle lobe. Which of the following organisms is most likely to be the cause of his symptoms?

A. Human immunodeficiency virus (HIV)
B. Escherichia coli
C. Chlamydia psittaci
D. Mycoplasma pneumoniae
E. Fusobacterium necrophorum

18. A patient returns from India with a productive cough. He also reported recent weight loss and night sweats. On examination cervical lymphadenopathy is found and described as being tender and tethered. What is the most useful investigation in confirming his underlying diagnosis?

A. Mantoux test
B. Interferon gamma release assay
C. Chest X-ray
D. Blood cultures
E. Sputum cultures stained with a Ziehl-Neelsen stain

19. A young woman who recently started medications to treat a tuberculosis infection accidentally fell pregnant, despite using the combined oral contraceptive pill. Which of the following medications is responsible for this?

A. Rifampicin
B. Isoniazid
C. Pyrazinamide
D. Ethambutol
E. Streptomycin

20. A young child is diagnosed with a Bordetella pertussis, by his general practitioner (GP). What form of prophylaxis should be given to his parents?

A. No prophylaxis is needed
B. Phenoxymethylpenicillin
C. Co-amoxiclav
D. Clarithromycin
E. Doxycycline

21. A lady who is 8 weeks pregnant presents to her general practitioner (GP) with dysuria and urinary frequency. A urine dip shows nitrites and leucocytes present in the urine. She also has a severe allergy to penicillin, which has previously resulted in anaphylaxis. Which of the following antibiotics should be prescribed?

A. Amoxicillin
B. Cephalexin
C. Nitrofurantoin
D. Trimethoprim
E. Gentamicin

22. A 30-year-old intravenous drug user presents to clinic for a check up. Which of the following should prompt a clinician into consenting him for a human immunodeficiency virus (HIV) test?

A. Shingles affecting only one dermatome
B. Fever and a new murmur
C. Severe new onset psoriasis
D. Cellulitis around needle marks
E. Tinea infection present in both inguinal regions

23. A patient who recently moved from the Africa to the United Kingdom presents to hospital with a fever. He reports having fevers, weight loss and night sweats for the past six months. On examination he has various dry warty hyperpigmented lesions on his skin, massive hepatosplenomegaly and cervical and inguinal lymphadenopathy. His neurological examination is unremarkable and he is alert throughout the consultation. His initial blood tests show a pancytopenia. Which of the following is the most likely underlying diagnosis?

A. Malaria
B. African trypanosomiasis
C. Toxoplasmosis
D. Visceral leishmaniasis
E. Human immunodeficiency virus (HIV)

24. A patient who recently returned from Sri Lanka 2 days ago presents to hospital with a fever. He describes having a headache, severe joint pains and feeling generally lethargic. On examination he has a temperature of 40 degrees Celsius, a widespread maculopapular rash and multiple mosquito bites on his ankles. His initial blood tests show low platelet count of $26 \times 10^9/L$ and deranged liver function tests, with a serum alanine aminotransferase (ALT) of 526 U/L. Which of the following is the most likely underlying diagnosis?

A   Influenza A
B.   Hepatitis A
C.   Dengue fever
D.   Malaria
E.   Typhoid

25. An 80-year-old female is admitted with pyrexia of unknown origin. She explains that she has lost 6 kilograms over the past 2 months and also noticed an increased frequency of her bowel motions. On examination of her fingernails she is found to have 7 splinter haemorrhages. Blood cultures are taken from three different sites. Which of the following organisms is most likely to be grown?

A.   Methicillin-resistant staphylococcus aureus
B.   Viridians Streptococcus
C.   Group A beta-haemolytic Streptococcus
D.   Streptococcus bovis
E.   Enterococcus

26. A gentleman with a new diagnosis of human immunodeficiency virus (HIV) is about to start antiretroviral therapy. His current CD4 count is 95 cells/μL. Which of the following medications should he commence along with his antiretroviral therapy?

A. Prednisolone
B. Sulfamethoxazole/trimethoprim
C. Doxycycline
D. Phenoxymethylpenicillin
E. Omeprazole

27. A 33-year-old lady has just returned from a holiday in Spain. She presents to the emergency department with a dry cough and worsening shortness of breath. She states this was preceded by a few days of malaise and arthralgia. She has a fever but all other observations are stable. Blood tests show a lymphocytopenia and hyponatraemia with a serum sodium of 125 mmol/L. Which of the following treatment regimes should be used to treat her hyponatraemia?

A. Fluid restriction
B. 3 litres of 0.9% saline given over 24 hours
C. 3 litres of 0.9% saline given over 24 hours and intravenous furosemide
D. 3 litres of 0.45% saline and 4% dextrose given over 24 hours
E. Oral fludrocortisone

28. A 32-year-old lady returns from Ghana with a fever. Following thick and thin blood films she is diagnosed with Falciparum malaria. She is started on intravenous quinine. Which of the following should be monitored meticulously following the initiation of her treatment?

A. Serum potassium
B. Serum sodium
C. Serum urea
D. Serum glucose
E. Quinine levels

29. A 34-year-old man is planning to travel to Nigeria for a month. He is prescribed some medication as a form of malaria prophylaxis. On returning to the United Kingdom he attends a doctor appointment complaining of an erythematous rash on his forearms, hands and face, all of which were exposed to sunlight during his travels. Which of the following drugs was he prescribed?

A. Mefloquine
B. Malarone
C. Chloroquine
D. Doxycycline
E. Proguanil

30. A 24-year-old woman presents with a history of vaginal discharge and has a vaginal swab taken. On wet microscopy stippled vaginal cells covered by gram-positive and gram-negative bacteria can be seen. Which of the following medications should be prescribed as first line treatment?

A. Azithromycin
B. Metronidazole
C. Intramuscular ceftriaxone
D. Doxycycline
E. Fluconazole

Infectious Diseases Answers

1. B
Trypanosoma cruzi

This patient has Chagas disease. It is caused by Trypanosoma cruzi, which can be found mainly in Latin America, and is transmitted by the Triatoma insect. An erythematous nodule forms at the bite site called a chagoma. Patients present with a fever, myalgia, unilateral conjunctivitis and hepatosplenomegaly. There is also muti-organ invasion. It can invade the myenteric plexus of the oesophagus and colon, causing both achalasia and a toxic megacolon respectively. It can also cause a dilated cardiomyopathy. This patient has developed both achalasia and a toxic megacolon.

Trypanosoma gambiense is a cause of African sleeping sickness, and is carried by the tsetse fly. It presents very non-specifically and causes headache, fever, rigors, and joint pains. It then progresses to cause meningoencephalitis, which presents with confusion, depression, convulsions and coma.

Leishmania braziliensis is a cause of mucocutaneous leishmaniasis. This presents with a primary skin lesion and progresses to cause lesions in the nose, pharynx, larynx and palate. These lesions can cause severe scarring.

Clostridium tetani is the cause of tetanus. It is a gram-positive anaerobic rod, which enters the body via deep cuts in the skin or mucosa. The bacteria release an exotoxin, which leads to a prodrome of fever and malaise. This is followed by muscle spasms and rigidity that classically present as lockjaw, hypertonic facial muscles and opisthotonus.

Polio is a picornavirus that is transmitted via the faecal-oral route. It initially causes a flu like prodrome, followed by a pre-paralytic phase consisting of fever, headache, vomiting and a unilateral tremor. Then some patients progress to the paralytic phase. This causes lower motor neurone signs, without any sensory signs.

2. D
Ivermectin

This patient has a Strongyloides stercoralis infection. This is a nematode, which enters the body via the skin and can cause a migrating urterica (cutaneous larva migrans). It travels to the lungs causing a pneumonitis, and also presents with abdominal pain and diarrhoea. In severe cases worms can take bacteria into the blood stream and cause septicaemia. A diagnosis can be made by stool microscopy. Ivermectin is an anti-parasitic drug, which can be used to treat Strongyloides stercoralis.

Metronidazole is an antibiotic used to treat anaerobic bacterial infections and also some parasitic infections such as Giardia lamblia and Entamoeba histolytica.

Amphotericin B is an anti-fungal drug given intravenously to treat severe systemic fungal infections such as cryptococcal meningitis and invasive aspergillosis.

Ceftriaxone is a third generation cephalosporin, which can be used to treat bacterial meningitis.

3. C
Praziquantel

This patient has become infected by Schistosomia haematobium, most likely from swimming in Lake Malawi. This is a trematode, which enters the bladder and causes frequency, haematuria, haematospermia and incontinence. If untreated there is scarring of the bladder and an increased risk of squamous cell carcinoma. It is the most common cause of squamous cell carcinoma of the bladder. Diagnosis can be made by microscopy of the urine showing the schistosomiasis eggs. Praziquantel is an anti-helmintic drug used treat Schistosomia haematobium.

Trimethoprim is an antibiotic that acts to inhibit the bacterial dihydrofolate reductase enzyme, and thus prevents DNA replication. It is often used as first line treatment for urinary tract infections.

Azithromycin is a macrolide antibiotic, and binds to the 50s subunit of the bacterial ribosome to prevent protein synthesis. It has a broad spectrum of activity but is most commonly used to treat Chlamydia trachomatis.

Cephalexin is a first generation cephalosporin, which is mainly active against gram-positive bacteria and disrupts the formation of the bacterial cell wall. It is used to treat urinary tract infections in pregnant women, when other drugs are contraindicated. However due to the risk of Clostridium difficile infections following cephalosporin use, it is rarely prescribed.

Fluconazole is an anti-fungal drug most commonly used to treat Candida infections. It can be given orally or intravenously if infections are severe, such as in an underlying human immunodeficiency virus (HIV) infection that has caused immunosuppression.

4. B
Ceftriaxone

Salmonella typhi is a gram-negative rod, which is transmitted by the faecal-oral route. It presents with a high fever, abdominal pain, constipation (which is more common than diarrhea), vomiting, a relative bradycardia, 'rose spots' and a dry cough. Complications include intestinal haemorrhage and perforation, abscesses and cholecystitis. The diagnosis is confirmed by culturing the bacteria. This can be difficult and bone marrow cultures often are the most sensitive, and may be required if the bacteria can't be grown in blood cultures. Due to resistance to multiple antibiotics, ceftriaxone is the first line treatment for Salmonella typhi. Fluoroquinolones, such as ciprofloxacin, may still be effective but growing resistance has lead to ceftriaxone becoming the first line treatment.

5. D
Campylobacter jejuni

Campylobacter jejuni infections often occur following the ingestion of undercooked chicken. Classically the worst symptom described is the stomach cramps. Patients also have bloody diarrhoea. Bloody diarrhoea makes the diagnosis more likely to be bacterial gastroenteritis than viral gastroenteritis. Campylobacter is a gram-negative spiral rod.

Other gram-negative rods that cause bacterial gastroenteritis include Escherichia coli, Salmonella enteritidis and Shigella dysenteriae and these are not spiral organisms. If antibiotics are required they are treated with ciprofloxacin.

Campylobacter jejuni is resistant to ciprofloxacin and therefore is treated with azithromycin. Two important complications of a Campylobacter jejuni infection are reactive arthritis and Guillain-Barre syndrome.

Bacillus cereus is a gram-positive rod. It produces endospores and therefore is protected against heat of less than 100 degrees Celsius. It has a short incubation time and causes nausea, vomiting and diarrhoea. Common culprits include re-heated milk, rice and infant formula.

Staphylococcus aureus is a gram-positive cocci, which produces an exotoxin. Therefore it has a short incubation time of 1–8 hours and symptoms of explosive vomiting and nausea start soon after ingesting the contaminated food. It is mainly found in contaminated dairy products.

6. A
Tinidazole

This patient has a Giardia lamblia infection. This is a protozoon, which is transmitted by contaminated water. The parasite attaches to the small intestine mucosa causing blunting of the villi and malabsorptive non-bloody diarrhoea. It causes steatorrhoea and weight loss. It classically has a long incubation period and therefore can be differentiated from other causes of infective diarrhoea. Tinidazole is the first line treatment for Giardia. Metronidazole can be used but it is thought that tinidazole is more effective.

Fluconazole is an anti-fungal drug, which can be used to treat candida and other fungal infections.

Co-trimoxazole is a combination of trimethoprim and sulfamethoxazole, which is most commonly used as prophylaxis against Pneumocystis jiroveci and Toxoplasma gondii in human immunodeficiency virus (HIV) positive patients.

Ciprofloxacin is a fluoroquinolone antibiotic, which is effective against most forms of bacterial gastroenteritis. However this is unlikely to be the cause of this patient's symptoms due to the long incubation period, long duration of symptoms and lack of bloody diarrhoea.

Erythromycin is a macrolide antibiotic. Azithromycin (another macrolide) is now used to treat gastroenteritis caused by Campylobacter jejuni, because it has become resistant to ciprofloxacin.

7. B
Cryptococcus neoformans

This patient has Cryptococcus meningitis. This is more common in immunocomprimised patients and it has a very insidious onset. Also it doesn't present with the classic features of meningitis. For example this patient is showing signs of photophobia but no neck stiffness. The bilateral sixth nerve palsy is a false localising sign that occurs when there is an increased intracranial pressure. Cryptococcus meningitis should be suspected in any immunocomprimised patient who becomes confused for a prolonged period of time. It can occur in any patient with a CD4 count < 100 cells/µL. It is diagnosed with an India ink stain of the cerebrospinal fluid (CSF) and treated with amphotericin B and flucytosine.

Toxoplasma infections can also occur in HIV positive patients with a CD4 count < 100 cells/µL. This is a parasitic infection that causes a posterior uveitis, encephalitis and focal neurological signs. It can lead to a raised intracranial pressure, due to inflammation, but this is more commonly seen in cryptococcal meningitis. Also imaging of the brain would classically show ring-enhancing lesions around the basal ganglia.

Mycobacterium tuberculosis can also cause meningitis, but would cause a positive IGRA test. Tuberculosis meningitis also has an insidious onset, and is diagnosed by use of a lumbar puncture. The cerebrospinal fluid would have a fibrin web formation, raised lymphocytes, raised protein and extremely low glucose levels.

Patients with HIV are at risk of disseminated cytomegalovirus infections, but these tend to occur at a CD4 count <50 cells/μL. They present with retinitis, colitis and meningoencephalitis.

8. D
Ciprofloxacin

A single dose of ciprofloxacin is now recommended as prophylaxis against meningitis. Previously it was rifampicin, but this would have been contraindicated in this patient due to her recent episode of jaundice and the hepatotoxic nature of rifampicin. Intramuscular ceftriaxone can be given as prophylaxis in pregnant women, but there is nothing in the history to suggest this lady is pregnant.

People who may require prophylaxis include household contacts, partners where a kissing relationship is present, and healthcare workers whose mouth or nose has been exposed directly to the infected patient (for example giving mouth to mouth during cardiopulmonary resuscitation).

Metronidazole can be given in combination with cefuroxime as prophylaxis prior to colorectal surgery. Clarithromycin is given as prophylaxis following exposure to pertussis.

9. D
Klebsiella pneumoniae

This patient has an abscess present in his lung, which can be diagnosed from the X-ray findings and his swinging fever. Klebsiella pneumoniae is an encapsulated, anaerobic, gram-negative rod, which is known to cause an atypical pneumonia. It can lead to abscess formation and classically causes green sputum. The foul smelling sputum indicates the causative organism is most likely to be anaerobic. Alcoholics and diabetic patients are more likely to be infected by Klebsiella pneumoniae.

Staphylococcus aureus and Pseudomonas are also causes of abscess formation.

Mycobacterium tuberculosis is likely to cause cavitating lesions, but these would be more likely to be present in the apices of the lungs, rather than the lower lobes.

Streptococcus pneumoniae doesn't classically cause abscess formation, but is by far the most common cause of pneumonia.

10. D
Diphtheria

This patient has a Corynebacterium diphtheria infection, which is a gram-positive rod. It is transmitted from human to human by air when an infected individual coughs or sneezes. In the United Kingdom it is not very common as children are now routinely vaccinated against diphtheria. Patients develop a high fever, cough, sore throat and grey or white plaques on their tonsils. They also have neck swelling because of cervical lymphadenopathy. Complications include myocarditis, neuropathy and low platelets that can lead to bleeding.

Rheumatic fever occurs following a Streptococcus pyogenes infection of the throat. It is an inflammatory condition that causes a fever, joint pains and a rash known as erythema marginatum. One of the long-term complications is rheumatic heart disease, whereby an autoimmune reaction occurs against the heart valves. It is the most common cause of mitral stenosis.

Measles presents with a high fever, conjunctivitis and a widespread rash. Complications include otitis media, pneumonia and subacute sclerosing panencephalitis.

Rubella presents with a fever, rash and lymphadenopathy. The main concern is that a rubella infection is teratogenic and can cause an intrauterine infection, which comprises of cardiac, cerebral, ophthalmic and auditory defects.

Polio is transmitted by the faecal-oral route and in many cases is asymptomatic or causes a minor infection. However rarely it can enter the central nervous system causing paralytic poliomyelitis.

11. E
Entamoeba histolytica

Entamoeba histolytica is a protozoa spread by the faecal-oral route. It causes colitis due to flask shaped ulcers in the colonic mucosa. The protozoa can then enter the portal vessels and travel to the liver. This patient has developed a liver abscess, hence the triad of a high swinging fever, right upper quadrant pain and jaundice. It is treated by use of metronidazole, and if an abscess forms it may require ultrasound-guided drainage.

Hepatitis A virus is spread by the faecal-oral route and it presents with a flu like prodrome consisting of fever, malaise arthralgia and anorexia, followed by jaundice and hepatomegaly. It does not cause a chronic hepatitis but can rarely cause acute fulminant hepatitis.

Cytomegalovirus infections in healthy individuals often just cause flu like symptoms. They can be problematic in immunocompromised patients causing retinitis, colitis and meningoencephalitis; and in pregnant women it can be vertically transmitted and cause fetal complications.

Mycobacterium tuberculosis is most likely to present with respiratory symptoms such as a cough, shortness of breath and haemoptysis. It can also infect other organs, but pulmonary tuberculosis is the most common.

Shistosoma mansoni infects the bladder causing haematuria, incontinence and haematospermia.

12. C
Ceftriaxone and ampicillin

This patient has meningitis caused by Listeria monocytogenes, which is a gram-positive bacillus. Those at risk include young children and the elderly. It presents like any other form of bacterial meningitis with fever, headache, meningism, photophobia and phonophobia. On performing a lumbar puncture gram-positive bacilli can be seen, along with a lymphocytosis. The treatment is to give both ceftriaxone and ampicillin.

Ceftriaxone alone would be given for all other causes of bacterial meningitis. These would show a neutrophilia in the CSF. Other bacterial causes include Neisseria meningitidis (encapsulated gram-negative diplococcus), Streptococcus pneumoniae (encapsulated gram-positive cocci) and rarely Haemophilus influenza (encapsulated gram-negative bacillus). Dexamethasone is only given with the first dose of antibiotics, and is used to reduce inflammation and reduce the likelihood of patients developing a sensorineural deafness, and is only used if pneumococcal meningitis is suspected.

Viral causes of meningitis include herpes simplex, varicella zoster and cytomegalovirus. The lumbar puncture and CSF analysis would show a lymphocytosis, raised protein and normal glucose level. Aciclovir can be used to treat viral meningitis caused by herpes simplex.

Rifampicin, isoniazid, pyrazinamide and ethambutol are used to treat tuberculosis meningitis. This would present with a more insidious onset and also cause the CSF to have formed a fibrin web, and show a lymphocytosis, raised protein, very low glucose and test positive for acid fast bacilli.

13. D
Haemophilus ducreyi

This patient has chancroid, which is the most common cause of sexually acquired genital ulcers in tropical countries. It is cause by Haemophilus ducreyi which is a gram-negative bacillus, and it presents with a painful ulcer. The ulcer has ragged borders and a yellow base. It can be treated with doxycycline.

Chlamydia trachomatis can be asymptomatic, but classically presents with discharge and dysuria. It can cause lymphogranuloma venerum, which would present with a painless ulcer and painful inguinal lymphadenopathy.

Treponema pallidum is a spirochete, which causes syphilis. Primary syphilis presents with a painless genital ulcer. The ulcer has well defined borders and is non-tender.

Klebsiella granulomatis causes granuloma inguinale, otherwise known as donovanosis. This presents with extensive painless red genital ulcers and inguinal node abscesses known as pseudobuboes. The ulcers can rupture and create fleshy oozing lesions, which allow the infection to spread.

Herpes simplex is a viral infection that is spread by skin contact. It causes painful ulcers and a viral prodrome, which includes fever, fatigue and arthralgia.

14. C
Atrioventricular block

This patient has a Borrelia burgdorfi infection (Lyme disease), which is spread by ticks. The rash being described is erythema migrans and occurs at the site where the patient is bitten by a tick. It can present with arthralgia, fatigue and fever. Its complications include meningitis, heart block, cranial nerve palsies (most commonly a facial nerve palsy) and neuropathy. Due to the lack of warning signs, sudden nature of collapse and rapid recovery, the cause of collapse is most likely to be a cardiac arrhythmia. Lyme disease is associated with atrioventricular block but not with aortic stenosis. If this patient had collapsed due to a seizure then meningitis would have been more likely.

Vasovagal collapse is more likely to be caused by some form of stimulus, and patients often describe feeling lightheaded and sounds becoming quieter just before the collapse.

In hypoglycemia patients would often describe sweating, anxiety, nausea and hunger prior to collapse.

15. C
Jarish-Herxheimer reaction

This patient has a secondary syphilis infection. A primary infection presents with a painless hard genital ulcer, and a secondary infection leads to a maculopapular rash. Upon treatment with antibiotics the Treponema pallidum releases endotoxins. This causes vasodilation, tachycardia and a fever. Also skin lesions can become enlarged. This Jarish-Herxheimer reaction is most common in secondary syphilis, and most dangerous in tertiary syphilis.

If a patient is given amoxicillin and has a concurrent Epstein-Barr virus (EBV) infection it causes a cross reaction and an amoxicillin induced exanthema. However an EBV infection would have presented with a fever, malaise and a sore throat.

Anaphylaxis can occur following administration of penicillins, but is more likely to cause stridor, dyspnea, angioedema, tachycardia and hypotension.

It is unlikely antibiotics would be contaminated with bacteria, but if sepsis did occur it would take longer to develop.

Reiter's syndrome is a reactive arthritis consisting of conjunctivitis, arthritis and urethritis. It occurs following infections such as Chlamydia and Campylobacter.

16. D
Leptospira interrogans

This patient has leptospirosis. Leptospira interrogans is transmitted in rat urine, so classically patients likely to contract it are sewage workers, farmers, and swimmers. It presents at first with a cough, chest pain, fever and myalgia. Another sign some patients present with is subconjunctival haemorrhages. Then after a few days patients either recover or develop Weil's disease, which includes uveitis, jaundice, renal failure and meningitis. If the infection is mild then doxycycline can be used, but if it is severe benzylpenicillin is required.

Legionella pneumonia is an atypical pneumonia, which is transmitted in water droplets. Therefore anyone exposed to a contaminated air conditioning unit is at risk. It presents with fever, cough and arthralgia.

Staphylococcus aureus is the most common cause of cellulitis. It can also cause toxic shock syndrome, which presents with shock, fever, confusion, desquamation of the skin and diarrhoea.

Bacillus anthracis is a gram-positive bacillus, which is spread by handling uncooked meats. Terrorists have also used it in the past as a biological weapon. It presents with a black pustule on the skin followed by oedema, fever and heptosplenomegaly. It rarely causes a pulmonary infection, which presents with flu like symptoms followed by pneumonia. It can cause a gastrointestinal infection due to consumption of infected meats, which presents with haematemisis, severe diarrhoea and anorexia.

Epstein-Barr virus (EBV) causes flu like symptoms, a sore throat, and malaise.

17. E
Fusobacterium necrophorum

This patient has developed Lemierre's syndrome, which is an infectious thrombophlebitis of the internal jugular vein, most commonly caused by Fusobacterium necrophorum (an anaerobic gram-negative bacteria). It presents with a fever, sore throat, neck pain and a cough. Complications include pulmonary abscesses and cavitations. Thrombosis of the internal jugular vein can be diagnosed by ultrasound, computed tomography (CT) or magnetic resonance imaging (MRI) scans, and requires treatment with anticoagulation. Fusobacterium necrophorum infections can be treated with beta-lactams, but patients often require additional anaerobic cover to ensure that other fusobacteria that may have varying degrees of resistance are treated, therefore it is common for metronidazole or clavulanic acid to be added to the antibiotic cover.

Chlamydia psittaci is an intracellular organism that can cause an atypical pneumonia and is transmitted to humans by infected birds. It can be treated with doxycycline.

Mycoplasma pneumoniae is another cause of an atypical pneumonia, which can rarely be complicated by erythema multiforme and Guillain-Barré syndrome. It can be treated with macrolide, tetracycline or fluoro-quinolone antibiotics.

Escherichia coli is a gram-negative rod, which is the most common cause of urinary tract infections.

HIV can present in various ways, but is not a cause of infectious thrombophlebitis and therefore is not the underlying cause in this case.

18. E
Sputum cultures stained with a Ziehl-Neelsen stain

Three early morning sputum samples are required for the diagnosis of active pulmonary tuberculosis. The Ziehl-Neelsen stain is used to identify Mycobacterium tuberculosis.

The matoux test would be positive in anyone who has had previous exposure to Mycobacterium tuberculosis or anyone who has had the Bacillus Calmette–Guérin (BCG) vaccine. It may also be positive in patients with exposure to non-tuberculosis mycobacterium, such as leprosy. Therefore it can be used as part of screening, but not to make a diagnosis.

Interferon gamma release assay (IGRA) is able to identify a current infection, but cannot tell whether that infection is latent or active. It measures the patient's white cell response to exposure to the Mycobacterium tuberculosis antigen.

Chest X-rays are very useful screening tools, but can't be used alone to make a diagnosis.

19. A
Rifampicin

Rifampicin is a P450 inducer and therefore it increases the liver metabolism of certain medications, including the combined oral contraceptive pill, thus making it less effective. Whilst women are taking rifampicin they should also use barrier methods of contraception, such as condoms.

Other side effects include hepatotoxicity and red secretions making both tears and urine red.

Isoniazid is a P450 inhibitor, and therefore wouldn't reduce the effect of the oral contraceptive pill. Its side effects include hepatotoxicity, peripheral neuropathy due to vitamin B6 deficiency, optic neuritis, drug induced lupus, agranulocytosis and aplastic anaemia.

Pyrazinamide can cause gout, due to raised levels of uric acid and is also hepatotoxic.

Ethambutol can cause an optic neuritis, which leads to loss of the colour vision first.

Streptomycin is an aminoglycoside and can cause nephrotoxicity and ototoxicity.

20. D
Clarithromycin

Clarithromycin is a macrolide that is used in both the treatment and prophylaxis of Bordetella pertussis (otherwise known as whooping cough). Prophylaxis is required for any household members, anyone who has been in close contact with the patient, or anyone who is at risk of a severe infection such as those that may be immunocompromised.

Phenoxymethylpenicillin (penicillin V) is given to patients who have had a splenectomy or asplenia (such as in sickle cell disease) as life long prophylaxis against pneumococcus.

Co-amoxiclav is given as a prophylactic antibiotic prior to a variety of surgeries including all gastrointestinal surgeries, and also following animal bites.

Doxycycline is a tetracycline and used in prophylaxis for malaria, Lyme disease and leptospirosis.

21. D
Nitrofurantoin

Normally patients who are pregnant and develop urinary tract infections (UTIs) are treated with either amoxicillin or cephalexin. However both these medications are contraindicated in this patient, because she is allergic to penicillin. Cephalosporins have cross-reactivity and 10% of patients with a penicillin allergy are also allergic to cephalosporins. Therefore unless it is absolutely necessary and there are no alternatives they shouldn't be prescribed.

Nitrofurantoin can also be used to treat UTIs, but should be avoided late in pregnancy as it can lead to a fetal haemolytic anaemia. This patient is still in her first trimester so nitrofurantoin is a safe option. Other side effects include peripheral neuropathy and pulmonary fibrosis.

Trimethoprim is contraindicated during the first trimester of pregnancy because of its activity against folate metabolism. It is teratogenic and can lead to miscarriage and fetal neural tube defects.

Gentamicin is an aminoglycoside and is used in the treatment of severe systemic bacterial infections such as infective endocarditis, septicaemia and peritonitis.

22. C
Severe new onset psoriasis

Psoriasis is a rash that often consists of multiple raised salmon coloured plaques on the extensor surfaces. It can be precipitated by many thing including drugs (beta-blockers and lithium) and also infections (Streptococcus and HIV). Therefore severe new onset psoriasis should prompt a HIV test.

Other signs that should also prompt a HIV test include: oral hairy leukoplakia, oral candida, karposi sarcoma, shingles across two or more dermatomes, widespread facial molluscum contagiosum, seborrheic dermatitis, cytomegalovirus retinitis and persistent generalised lymphadenopathy.

Shingles affecting only one dermatome isn't a sign of immuno-suppression. A fever and a new murmur should prompt investigation for infective endocarditis. Cellulitis around needle marks often occurs if intravenous drug users are using contaminated needles. It is relatively common and doesn't require a HIV test. Tinea is a fungal infection also known as ringworm. It occurs in warm, moist areas of the body such as in the groin and in between skin folds. It is a common condition and is not associated with a HIV infection.

23. D
Visceral leishmaniasis

Visceral leishmaniasis (also known as Kala-azar) is the second most deadly parasitic infection in the world following malaria. It is transmitted by sandflies and occurs across Africa, Asia, South America and Europe. The main causes are Leishmania donovani and Leishmania chagasai. It has a prolonged incubation period of months or even years in some cases. It presents with skin lesions, fevers, night sweats, burning feet, arthralgia, splenomegaly, hepatomegaly and lymphadenopathy. Blood tests show a pancytopenia and hypergammaglobulinemia. Diagnosis can be made by microscopic examination of the lymph nodes, spleen or bone marrow.

Malaria is the main differential for patients returning from Africa with a fever. However it doesn't cause a rash or lymphadenopathy. Malaria would present with a short history of a fevers and rigors. Patients can also develop jaundice and hepatosplenomegaly. The diagnosis is confirmed using serial thick and thin blood films.

Toxoplasma infections are often asymptomatic but can be severe in immunocompromised individuals. In such patients toxoplasmosis can lead to encephalitis, focal neurological signs and seizures.

African trypanosomiasis is also known as sleeping sickness and is caused by Trypanosoma gambiense and Trypanosoma rhodesiense, which are both transmitted by the tsetse fly. It presents with a tender subcutaneous nodule at the site of infection. The disease then has two stages. Initially patients are non-specifically unwell with fevers, rashes, joint pains and may develop Winterbottom's sign, which is a palpable posterior cervical lymph node. Following this patients develop neurological sequel with seizures, agitation, confusion, hypersomnolence and eventually develop a coma.

24. C
Dengue fever

Dengue fever is a mosquito-borne tropical disease caused by the dengue virus. Symptoms typically begin between 3 and 14 days after the mostquito bite. Symptoms include high fevers, headaches, nausea, joint pains and a rash. Typically the blood tests will show low platelets and a transaminitis. Dengue is very common across the whole of South East Asia. The diagnosis is confirmed by serology and the treatment is supportive.

Hepatitis A is also common across the whole of Asia, Africa and South America. It is transmitted by the faecal-oral route and symptoms typically appear 2 to 6 weeks after the initial infection. It causes an acute hepatitis and patients often present with fever, nausea, fatigue and jaundice. The diagnosis is confirmed by serology. Treatment is supportive, but there is also a vaccine that should be given to patients to before they travel. Hepatitis A doesn't cause a rash, and therefore this patient's presentation is more in keeping with dengue fever.

Sri Lanka is not an area where malaria is found, and malaria wouldn't present with a rash. Malaria would present with a short history of a fevers and rigors. Patients can also develop jaundice and hepatosplenomegaly.

Typhoid is caused by Salmonella typhi and is transmitted by the faecal-oral route. It can also be found across South East Asia, and presents with a high fever, abdominal pain, constipation (which is more common than diarrhea), vomiting, a relative bradycardia, 'rose spots' and a dry cough.

Influenza A is a viral respiratory tract infection spread by water droplets. It presents with a fever, headache, malaise, joint pains, a cough and shortness of breath.

25. D
Streptococcus bovis

This patient has developed infective endocarditis. This is likely because of her unexplained fever and 7 splinter haemorrhages (>5 are seen as abnormal). Splinter haemorrhages occur as a result of immune complex deposition in the nail bed vessels. She also has an underlying diagnosis of colorectal cancer. This is likely because of her age, weight loss and diarrhoea occurring for the last two months. Any patient over 60 years old who has a change in bowel habit for more than 6 weeks requires urgent investigation for colorectal cancer. Colorectal cancer is associated with a Streptococcus bovis infective endocarditis, and therefore this is the most likely organism to be grown in the blood cultures.

Methicillin-resistant staphylococcus aureus would be most likely if this patient had just undergone a valve replacement.

Viridians Streptococcus is one of the most common causes of infective endocarditis and is classically associated with dental procedures.

Enterococcus is associated with gastrointestinal or genitourinary tract surgery and also prolonged urinary tract infections.

Group A beta-haemolytic Streptococcus is also known as Streptococcus pyogenes. This doesn't cause infective endocarditis but does cause rheumatic fever.

26. B
Sulfamethoxazole/trimethoprim

This gentleman has a low CD4 count and therefore should be prescribed prophylactic sulfamethoxazole/trimethoprim (also known as co-trimoxazole) to prevent both Pneumocystis jirovecii and Toxoplasma gondii infections. Prophylactic co-trimoxazole is routinely given to anyone with HIV that has a CD4 count of less than 200 cells/μL. Once the CD4 count is less than 200 cells/μL the patient is at risk of Pneumocystis jirovecii infections and once it is less than 100 cells/μL the patient is at risk of Toxoplasma gondii infections.

Doxycycline is used as malaria prophylaxis, and phenoxymethylpenicillin (also known as penicillin V) is used as prophylaxis against infections in patients that have hyposplenism or a splenectomy.

27. A
Fluid restriction

This lady has developed syndrome of inappropriate antidiuretic hormone (ADH) secretion (SIADH) from a Legionella pneumonia. She has just returned from Spain, and air conditioning units in hotels can predispose people to Legionella pneumophila infections. Furthermore she has all the symptoms of an atypical pneumonia, which include a prodrome of malaise and arthralgia followed by a dry cough. Legionnaires' disease is known to cause a lymphopenia.

SIADH has many causes such as infections (meningnoencephalitis, brain abscesses), malignancy (small cell lung cancer), drugs (selective serotonin reuptake inhibitors (SSRIs), carbamazepine) and many more. For a diagnosis of SIADH, patients must be euvolaemic, hyponatraemic, with concentrated urine with an osmolality >500 mOsm/kg and urine sodium >20 mmol/L.

Treatment includes treating the underlying cause, fluid restriction, and if really severe use of vaptans (vasopressin receptor antagonists) or demeclocycline (a tetracycline antibiotic which has a side effect of inducing nephrogenic diabetes insipidus).

Oral fludrocortisone is a synthetic mineralocorticoid and aldosterone receptor agonist that causes salt and fluid retention. It is used in Addison's disease and postural hypotension.

Giving fluids in this patient is likely to worsen the hyponatraemia and therefore all options involving fluids are incorrect.

28. D
Serum glucose

Quinine is used to treat Plasmodium falciparum malaria. Its side effects include hypoglycemia, tinnitus, vertigo; blood disorders such as thrombocytopenia and disseminated intravascular coagulation (DIC) and long QT syndrome. Therefore these patients require both glucose and cardiac monitoring. Quinine doesn't require its levels to be monitored. Quinine has been used in the past to treat leg cramps, however due to its side effects it is no longer recommended.

29. D
Doxycycline

Doxycycline is a tetracycline antibiotic, which is used as prophylaxis in areas of chloroquine resistance. Its main side effects are teratogenicity, oseophagitis and a photosensitive rash. This patient has described a rash only occurring in areas that would have been exposed to the sun, making a photosensitive rash the most likely cause. The rash disappears on discontinuation of the drug.

Mefloquine is a form of malaria prophylaxis used in areas with high risk of chloroquine resistant Plasmodium falciparum. However it is known to cause neuropsychiatric reactions (such as anxiety, depression, hallucinations and psychosis).

Malarone is a combination of atovaquone and proguanil. Its main side effects are abdominal pain, nausea and headaches. Proguanil can be used alone and can cause gastrointestinal side effects such as diarrhoea.

Chloroquine is used as prophylaxis where there is a low risk of chloroquine resistance, but is no longer used as treatment for Plasmodium falciparum malaria. Its side effects include lowering the seizure threshold and visual disturbance due to retinopathy.

30. B
Metronidazole

This patient has developed bacterial vaginosis. This occurs due to an increase in the vaginal pH and a change in the natural flora of the vagina. There is overgrowth of bacteria such as Gardnerella vaginalis, Mycoplasma hominis, and Peptostreptococci. These replace the lactobacilli that are normally present, and cause a foul smelling fishy discharge. The main risk factor for bacterial vaginosis is genital washing. The cells seen on wet microscopy are 'clue cells' and are diagnostic of bacterial vaginosis. The first line treatment is metronidazole.

Azithromycin is used to treat Chlamydia trachomatis, and intramuscular ceftriaxone is used to treat Neisseria gonorrhoea infections. Both infections are diagnosed by use of a nucleic acid amplification tests. Current guidelines state that patents that are diagnosed with one of these infections should be treated for both. Both infections can be asymptomatic or present with discharge and dysuria.

Doxycycline can also be used to treat Chlamydia trachomatis infections, especially those that result in a proctitis or cause lymphogranuloma venereum. Lymphogranuloma venerum presents with a painless genital ulcer, followed by painful inguinal lymphadenopathy and eventually patients can develop a proctocolitis.

Fluconazole is used to treat thrush (vaginal candida infections). This presents with a curd like discharge and puritis. Risk factors include diabetes mellitus, pregnancy, broad-spectrum antibiotics and use of the oral contraceptive pill. Microscopy would show strings of mycelium and oval spores. Topical clotrimazole can be used along with oral fluconazole.

Neurology Questions

1. A middle aged man presents to clinic with a history of severe headaches. The pain is unilateral, periocular and associated with lacrimation and rhinorrhea. The headaches don't appear to be precipitated by anything but occur at exactly 3pm every day. Which of the following drugs could be used as prophylaxis to prevent these headaches occuring?

A. Sumatriptan
B. Verapamil
C. Intranasal lidocaine
D. Gabapentin
E. High flow oxygen therapy

2. A 56-year-old man with a history of bipolar affective disorder, controlled by lithium, presents to his general practitioner (GP) with a painful red swelling in his first metatarsophalangeal joint. He is apyrexial and systemically well. He is prescribed some medication by the GP. Three days later he presents to hospital with diarrhoea, vomiting, a course tremor and reduced consciousness. Which of the following drugs was prescribed by the GP?

A. Paracetamol
B. Indometacin
C. Codeine phosphate
D. Colchicine
E. Clindamycin

3. A 35-year-old woman being treated for multiple sclerosis tests positive for a latent JC virus infection. Which of the following treatments is contraindicated in this patient?

A. Methylprednisolone
B. Interferon-1β
C. Azathioprine
D. Natalizumab
E. Glatiramer

4. A 45-year-old woman with a previous history of well controlled myasthenia gravis presents to hospital with a fever and malaise. On examination it is noticed that she has a new pan systolic murmur heard loudest at the apex. Following four days of intravenous antibiotics she develops a complex ophthalmoplegia, bilateral ptosis and proximal muscle weakness that is worse by the end of the day. Which antibiotic is responsible for her new symptoms?

A. Benzylpenicillin
B. Flucloxacillin
C. Vancomycin
D. Gentamicin
E. Clindamycin

5. A young man presents to his general practitioner (GP) 3 months after a traumatic road traffic accident with a severe neuropathic burning pain in his right leg. The GP prescribes him with some medication to relieve his pain. A week later he returns to his GP with an extremely painful red eye, nausea and vomiting. He describes seeing halos around bright lights and on examination his GP notices a hazy cornea in the affected eye. Which medication was this patient prescribed one week ago?

A. Gabapentin
B. Amitriptyline
C. Duloxetine
D. Carbamazepine
E. Tramadol

6. A 45-year-old man presents to hospital with a severe sudden onset occipital headache, nausea, vomiting, neck stiffness and photophobia. On examination he is found to have a left sided hemiparesis. What is the most appropriate next step in this patient's management plan?

A. 300 mg of aspirin
B. Alteplase
C. Nimodipine
D. Computed tomography (CT) scan of the head
E. Lumbar puncture

7. A patient presents to hospital with an ascending weakness that began in his legs and has spread to the rest of his body. On examination it is found that he has a complex ophthalmoplegia, ataxia and areflexia. Which of the following antibodies are likely to be found in the patient's serum?

A. Anti-GM1
B. Anti-GQ1b
C. Anti-MuSK
D. Anti-Ach receptor
E. Anti-NMO

8. A patient with a previous history of paroxysmal nocturnal haemo-globinurea presents to clinic with a headache, loss of sensation on the whole of the right side of his face, and also diplopia caused by looking to the right. These symptoms had progressively worsened over the last few weeks. A magnetic resonance venogram was used to confirm the diagnosis. What is the most likely explanation for this patient's symptoms?

A. Subdural haemorrhage
B. Lateral medullary infarction
C. Parietal lobe astrocytoma
D. Subarachnoid hemorrhage
E. Inferior petrosal sinus thrombus

9. An elderly man presents to a neurology clinic with a gradual onset of weakness. This began six months ago and originally only affected his hands, but the weakness has now spread to his shoulders and legs. On examination he has florid fasciculations that can be seen in both arms, wasting and flaccid weakness in his right arm and spastic weakness in his left leg. He also has hyperreflexia in both knees. His sensory exam is completely normal. What is the most likely underlying diagnosis?

A. Amyotrophic lateral sclerosis
B. Guillain-Barre syndrome
C. Chronic inflammatory demyelinating polyneuropathy
D. Multiple sclerosis
E. Myasthenia gravis

10. An elderly patient who was recently diagnosed with Parkinson's disease has been prescribed L-3,4-dihydroxyphenylalanine (L-DOPA). She is also prescribed carbidopa, and was told by her doctor that carbidopa is used to prevent the side effects that can be caused by L-DOPA. Which of the following side effects of L-DOPA can be prevented by carbidopa?

A. Hallucinations
B. Insomnia
C. Vivid dreams
D. Dyskinesia
E. Hypotension

11. An 88-year-old woman presents to clinic with a headache and bilateral leg weakness. On examination she is found to have bilateral brisk knee jerks and upward going plantars. What is the most likely underlying diagnosis?

A. Anterior spinal artery syndrome
B. Multiple sclerosis
C. Glioblastoma multiforme of the left frontal lobe
D. Chronic inflammatory demyelinating polyneuropathy
E. Meningioma of the falx cerbri

12. A 22-year-old woman presents to hospital following a fall and loss of consciousness. She described feeling confused and tired after waking. She also stated she had weakness in her left arm and leg. She was admitted to hospital and remained there till her symptoms fully resolved 12 hours later. What is the underlying cause of her symptoms?

A. Transient ischaemic attack
B. Ischaemic stroke
C. Multiple sclerosis
D. Migraine
E. Epilepsy

13. A patient presents with diplopia. On examination the left pupil is unreactive to light, there is ipsilateral ptosis and the eye is fixed looking downwards and laterally. What is the underlying diagnosis?

A. Diabetic neuropathy
B. Horner's syndrome
C. Argyll Robertson pupil
D. Posterior communicating artery aneurysm
E. Lacunar infarction

14. A patient presents with weakness in his left arm and left leg. He has ptosis of his right eye and the eye is deviated downwards and to the right. It was concluded that this patient had an ischaemic stroke. What was the most likely location of his stroke?

A. Basilar artery
B. Left middle cerebral artery
C. Right lateral medulla
D. Right midbrain
E. Right posterior limb of the internal capsule

15. A 15-year-old boy presents to clinic with increasing fatigue. On examination it is found that the patient has an ataxic gait, nystagums, absent knee reflexes and upward going plantars. He also reveals that he is currently being seeing a cardiologist, due to recurrent episodes of syncope. What is the most likely underlying diagnosis?

A. Ataxic telangiectasia
B. Congenital syphilis infection
C. Subacute combined degeneration of the spinal cord
D. Friedreich's ataxia
E. Neuromyelitis optica

16. A 75-year-old man is described as having recurrent hallucinations and fluctuating cognition. In the clinic you notice that he has a soft monotonous voice and an expressionless face. Which of the following proteins is responsible for the pathology in the underlying diagnosis?

A. α-synuclein
B. β-amyloid
C. Tau
D. TAR DNA-binding protein 43 (TDP-43)
E. Superoxide dismutase 1 (SOD1)

17. A 61-year-old patient diagnosed with amyotrophic lateral sclerosis is brought into clinic by her concerned husband. He states that over the past few months she has become increasingly apathetic about her condition and also appears to have lost her ability to empathise with those around her. What is the most likely underlying cause of her recent change in personality?

A. Alzheimer's disease
B. Frontotemporal dementia
C. Depression
D. Delirium
E. Side effect of riluzole

18. A patient has two seizures and was subsequently started on an antiepileptic drug. He is seizure free for three weeks, and his epilepsy improves. However he then begins to develop seizures again, despite him being fully compliant with his medication. Which of the following drugs was he prescribed?

A. Carbamazepine
B. Sodium valproate
C. Lamotrigine
D. Ethosuximide
E. Diazepam

19. A 40-year-old male presents with increasing memory loss and recent episodes of diarrhoea. When speaking to him it becomes apparent that he is feeling low, tired and has had trouble sleeping recently. He has also lost his appetite. On examination there is nothing of note except for an erythematous rash around his neck. What is the most likely underlying diagnosis?

A. Whipple's disease
B. Toxoplasmosis
C. Neurosyphilis
D. Pellegra
E. Thiamine deficiency

20. A 21-year-old female asthmatic who is currently trying to conceive attends her general practice for the fourth time in three weeks complaining of a headache. She described it as a unilateral throbbing headache associated with photophobia and vomiting. Which of the following should be prescribed as long-term prophylaxis?

A. Sumatriptan
B. Propranolol
C. Topiramate
D. Amitriptyline
E. Paracetamol and metoclopramide

21. A 60-year-old male presents to hospital with new onset unilateral deafness and a right sided facial droop. On examination it is found that the Weber test lateralises to the left ear and when performing the Rinne test on the both the left and right ears the vibration could be heard loudest in front of both ears, rather than when the tuning fork was pressed against the mastoid process. Which of the following tests should be carried out to confirm the underlying diagnosis?

A. Audiometry
B. Otoscopy
C. Magnetic resonance imaging (MRI) scan of the head
D. Facial nerve electromyography
E. Serum calcium, phosphate and alkaline phosphatase (ALP)

22. A 75-year-old male is diagnosed with dementia following a 6 month history of worsening memory. He is due to be started on done-pezil, to slow the progression of his condition. Which of the following investigations should be carried out before starting the new drug?

A. Full blood count (FBC)
B. Urea and electrolytes (U&Es)
C. Liver function tests (LFTs)
D. Electrocardiogram (ECG)
E. Chest X-ray

23. A 35-year-old presents to hospital with sudden onset left sided facial droop. She is unable to raise her eyebrow on the left side of her face. There is no other weakness found on examination of her upper and lower limbs, and no sensory loss. Which of the following investigations should occur next?

A. Computed tomography (CT) scan of the head
B. Facial nerve electromyography (EMG)
C. Visual acuity using a Snellen chart
D. Otoscopy
E. Audiometry

24. A 40-year-old male presents with a 4-week history non-specific generalised muscle pains and weakness. He also reports sporadic fasciculations. On examination there is no sensory loss but the doctor notices a blue tinge along the patient's gums. The weakness is worse in his left leg and as part of his work-up an X-ray of his knee is requested and shows dense metaphyseal lines. What is the most likely underlying diagnosis?

A. Chronic inflammatory demyelinating polyneuropathy
B. Vitamin B12 deficiency
C. Side effects from a previous chemotherapy regime
D. Lead poisoning
E. Acute intermittent porphyria

25. A 65-year-old man is admitted to hospital following a suspected stoke. As part of his workup he has a full neurological examination, which shows a right hemiplegia with forehead sparing and no sensory loss. Which of the following areas is most likely to have been affected by the stroke?

A. Anterior cerebral artery
B. Middle cerebral artery
C. Posterior cerebral artery
D. Posterior limb of the internal capsule
E. Ventral posterolateral nucleus of the thalamus

26. A 70-year-old lady with a smoking history of 60 pack years is admitted following a stroke. On examination she is found to have sensory loss of pain and temperature on the left side of her face, and on the right side of her torso. She also has partial ptosis, miosis, and anhidrosis on the left side of her face. Which of the following arteries is most likely to have been affected by the stroke?

A. Posterior inferior cerebellar artery
B. Basilar artery
C. Anterior spinal artery
D. Middle cerebral artery
E. Lenticulostriate artery

27. A 30-year-old man is brought into hospital at 2am on a Sunday morning following a mechanical fall on his way back from the pub. As he fell he knocked his head on the pavement but didn't lose consciousness. A concerned friend who brought him into hospital stated that he slipped on a frozen puddle. Which of the following aspects of his history or examination would lead you to requesting an urgent computed tomography (CT) scan of his head?

A. Five minutes after the fall his Glasgow Coma Scale (GCS) score was 14
B. He vomited once following the injury
C. He is currently taking aspirin and clopidogrel
D. Otoscopy revealed evidence of blood in the middle ear
E. As he fell he bit the tip of his tongue

28. A 50-year-old man presents complaining of episodes of dizziness that last up to a few hours. He states that when it occurs the room appears to spin horizontally around him and a buzzing noise is heard in his left ear. He has also found that he can't hear anything in his left ear during these episodes. Which of the following can be given as prophylaxis for these attacks?

A. Prochlorperazine
B. Betahistine
C. Cinnarizine
D. Metoclopramide
E. Instructions on how to perform an Epley manoeuvre

29. An 80-year-old male with dementia and a history of alcoholism, has been admitted to hospital 6 times over the past 2 months following falls. His wife who believes he has become more forgetful and drowsy over the past 2 weeks takes him to see his general practitioner (GP). At his most recent check up 3 weeks ago his abbreviated mental test score (AMTS) was 8, whereas now it is 5. What is the most likely diagnosis?

A. Rapidly progressing Alzheimer's disease
B. Vascular dementia and a recent ischaemic stroke
C. Subdural haemorrhage
D. Depression
E. Korsakoff's syndrome

30. An obese 34-year-old female, presents with a generalised headache, which is worse on leading forwards and sneezing. On examination she is found to have bilateral papillodema, blurred vision but no photophobia. She currently takes a number of medications. Which of the following drugs could be responsible for her headache?

A. Glyceryl trinitrate (GTN) spray
B. Isotretinoin
C. Codeine phosphate
D. Caffeine
E. Nifedipine

Neurology Answers

1. B
Verapamil

This patient has cluster headaches, which are severe, unilateral headaches accompanied by autonomic symptoms such as lacrimation and rhinorrhea. They classically occur at the same time every day. Verapamil is a non-dihydropyridine calcium channel blocker and can be used as prophylaxis to prevent cluster headaches occurring.

In the acute setting high flow oxygen, sumatriptan and intranasal lidocaine can be used. Sumatriptan belongs to the triptan class and is a 5-hydroxytryptamine (5HT) receptor agonist that acts by causing vasoconstriction. It decreases the activity of the trigeminal nerve, which is over stimulated in cluster headaches. Triptans can also be used to treat migraines as they reduce the vascular inflammation that is thought to occur during a migraine. These drugs are only used acutely and therefore verapamil would be most suitable as a prophylactic agent.

Gabapentin is an anticonvulsant medication, which is mainly used to treat neuropathic pain but can also be used to prevent seizures. It doesn't have a role in treating cluster headaches.

2. B
Indometacin

This patient had gout and was prescribed indometacin, which is a strong non-steroidal anti-inflammatory drug (NSAID), as treatment. He is also currently on lithium for bipolar affective disorder, and the concurrent prescription of an NSAID caused lithium toxicity. Other drugs that can cause lithium toxicity are diuretics, angiotensin converting enzyme (ACE) inhibitors and angiotensin receptor II blockers. Any condition that lowers the serum sodium can also lead to lithium toxicity. These patients are advised to avoid a low salt diet and to seek medical help if they develop vomiting or diarrhoea. Lithium toxicity presents with diarrhoea, vomiting, cerebellar signs, a course tremor, seizures and renal failure. Treatment is to give intravenous saline and if toxicity is severe haemodialysis is used.

Lithium can cause many side effects. Short-term side effects include oedema, weight gain and a metallic taste in the mouth. Long-term side effects include nephrogenic diabetes insipidus, chronic kidney disease, hypothyroidism, acne, psoriasis, and a fine tremor.

The other drug listed that can be used to treat gout is colchicine. In this scenario, colchicine would have been a better option because it doesn't interact with lithium.

Paracetamol and codeine phosphate are both painkillers, but are not used to treat acute gout.

Clindamycin is an antibiotic, which can used to treat Staphylococcal infections, but is not commonly used as it can result in Clostridium difficle infections.

3. D
Natalizumab

Natalizumab is a monoclonal antibody against α4-integrin (which is normally used to allow white blood cells to cross the blood brain barrier). This is used in multiple sclerosis to reduce the number of relapses.

However if patients are carriers of the JC virus the white blood cells can't enter the brain to fight the infection and thus it leads to progressive multifocal leukoencephalopathy, which is often fatal.

Interferon-1β is also used to reduce relapses and reduces the number of brain lesions that can be seen on magnetic resonance imaging (MRI). Glatriamer is an alternative drug to interferon-1β.

Methylprednisolone is used in the acute setting to shorten the duration of the relapse, but it doesn't have any effect on long-term prognosis.

4. D
Gentamicin

This patient has been brought in with infective endocarditis (hence her fever and new murmur). However she also has an underlying diagnosis of myasthenia gravis. This is evident by the worsening symptoms, which she develops following treatment. Myasthenia gravis classically presents with ptosis, a complex ophthalmoplegia and increasing muscle fatigue that starts by affecting the facial muscles, followed by the neck and limbs. A myasthenic crisis can be precipitated by gentamicin.

Other drugs that can precipitate a crisis include opiates, tetracyclines, quinine and beta-blockers. Other precipitants include pregnancy, hypokalaemia, and exercise. The other antibiotics listed don't have any affect on myasthenia gravis.

5. B
Amitriptyline

This patient has acute angle glaucoma. This presents with a painful red eye, nausea and vomiting, a hazy cornea and dilated pupil. It is caused by an acute increase in intraocular pressure due to a build up of fluid in the eye. This is due to the fixed dilated pupil blocking the drainage of the intraocular fluid.

Therefore any drug that causes dilation of the pupils can precipitate acute angle glaucoma. Tricyclic antidepressants have antimuscarinic properties and cause pupil dilation. Other drugs with antimuscarinic properties include oxybutinin, antipsychotics and antihistamines. Drugs that also dilate the pupils through other mechanisms include beta-agonists such as salbutamol, and recreational stimulants such as cocaine.

Gabapentin is an anti-epileptic drug that is now more commonly used to treat neuropathic pain.

Duloxetine is a serotonin-norepinephrine reuptake inhibitor (SNRI), which is used to treat patients who have a diabetic neuropathy.

Carbamazepine is an anti-epileptic drug, which is effective at treating trigeminal neuralgia, neuropathic pain and mania.

Tramadol is an opioid used to treat pain.

6. C
Computed tomography (CT) scan of the head

This patient is having a subarachnoid haemorrhage, which is caused by rupture of saccular/berry aneurysms or arteriovenous malformations. This causes a build up of blood between the arachnoid and pia meningeal layers. It presents with a 'thunderclap' headache, meningism due to meningeal irritation and can also cause focal neurology. Urgent confirmation of the diagnosis is made by use of a CT scan of the head. Evidence on the scan includes blood around the circle of Willis, in the basal cisterns, the lateral ventricles and in the 4th ventricle. If the CT scan is negative then a lumber puncture can be performed 12 hours after the onset of the headache. Blood present in the cerebrospinal fluid (CSF) becomes xanthochromic (yellow) after a few hours, due to the breakdown of the red blood cells to form bilirubin. A CT scan must always be carried out first; to ensure the intracranial pressure is not raised.

9"x6"
b3668_01-Cardiology.indd 3
b3668   320 Single Best Answer Questions for Final Year Medical Students
23-Aug-19 6:

Neurology Answers   **191**

Three hundred milligrams of aspirin would be given in a non-haemorrhagic stroke, or in a transient ischaemic attack. Alteplase is used as thrombolytic treatment in an ischaemic stroke, and must be administered within 4.5 hours of the onset of symptoms. Past this point the risks of thrombolysis outweigh the benefits.

Nimodipine is a calcium channel antagonist that is used in a subarachnoid haemorrhage to reduce the chance of vasospasm. Vasospasm can occur due to the presence of blood in the subarachnoid space, causing irritation of the blood vessels. This can result in a secondary ischaemic stroke.

7. B
Anti-GQ1b

This patient has developed Miller Fisher syndrome, and has presented with the classic triad of ophthalmoplegia, ataxia and areflexia. Miller Fisher syndrome is a varient of Guillian-Barre syndrome, and weakness of the extra-ocular muscles is more pronounced. It is diagnosed by the presence of anti-GQ1b antibodies.

Anti-GM1 antibodies are found in Guillian-Barre syndrome. This is a condition that presents with ascending weakness and areflexia. It is an autoimmune disease caused by demyelination of the lower motor neurones. It can be precipitated by infections such as Campylobacter jejuni, Mycoplasma pneumoniae, cytomegalovirus and Epstein-Barr virus. In the acute phase it can cause life threatening respiratory failure.

Anti-Ach receptor and Anti-MuSK antibodies are found in myasthenia gravis, which would present with progressive muscle weakness that worsens throughout the day. It starts by affecting the eyes, causing a complex ophthalmoplegia and then moves downwards to affect the proximal muscles. It wouldn't cause areflexia or ataxia.

Anti-NMO antibodies are found in neuromyelitis optica (NMO), otherwise known as Devic's syndrome, which causes the autoimmune demyelination of the central nervous system. It presents with optic neuritis and transverse myelitis. It can be differentiated from multiple sclerosis by the presence of anti-NMO antibodies and absence of cerebrospinal fluid (CSF) oligoclonal bands.

8. E
Inferior petrosal sinus thrombus

This patient is hypercoagulable due to their underlying diagnosis of paroxysmal nocturnal haemoglobinurea. This and the fact that a magnetic resonance venogram was used to confirm the diagnosis make a venous thrombus the most likely cause of this patient's symptoms. An inferior petrosal sinus thrombus can cause a fifth and sixth nerve palsy. A fifth nerve palsy would cause the loss of sensation described and a sixth nerve palsy would prevent the lateral movement of the eye leading to diplopia. This condition is also known as Gradenigo's syndrome.

A subdural haemorrhage would present with a headache, fluctuating consciousness, drowsiness and personality change. Risk factors include dementia, alcoholism and anticoagulation.

A lateral medullary infarction is also known as Wallenberg's syndrome, and is due to occlusion of the posterior inferior cerebellar artery. It causes ipsilateral Horner's syndrome, cerebellar signs and loss of pain and temperature sensation on the face, and contralateral loss of pain and temperature sensation on the torso.

Parietal lobe astrocytoma would present with hemisensory loss and loss of two point discrimination. If it affected the dominant hemisphere it could cause Gerstmann's syndrome, which comprises of finger agnosia, agraphia, alexia and acalculia. If it affects the non-dominant hemisphere it could cause contralateral side neglect.

A subarachnoid haemorrhage would present with a severe sudden onset occipital headache, neck stiffness, photophobia and phonophobia. It is caused by rupture of a saccular/berry aneurysm or arteriovenous malformation, leading to blood building up between the arachnoid and pia meningeal layers.

9. A
Amyotrophic lateral sclerosis

This patient is has a mixture of upper and lower motor neurone signs, with no sensory deficit. Upper motor neurone signs include spasticity caused by increased tone, weakness, hyperreflexia and upward going plantars, while lower motor neurone signs include wasting, fasciculations, flaccid weakness due to reduced tone and hyporeflexia/areflexia. The mixture of upper and lower motor neurone signs with no sensory defect makes amyotrophic lateral sclerosis the most likely diagnosis.

Guillain-Barre syndrome is caused by autoimmune destruction of the peripheral nervous system. It can occur following certain infections such as Campylobacter jejuni, Mycoplasma pneumoniae, cytomegalovirus and Epstein-Barr virus. It presents with an ascending weakness that begins at the feet and rapidly spreads to the rest of the body. It causes changes in sensation, pain and lower motor neurone signs as both the peripheral sensory and motor neurones are affected.

Chronic inflammatory demyelinating polyneuropathy (CIDP) is an acquired immune-mediated inflammatory disorder of the peripheral nervous system, which also presents with both sensory and lower motor neurone signs but has a more insidious onset than Guillain-Barre syndrome.

Multiple sclerosis is caused by demyelination of the central nervous system causing upper motor neurone signs and most commonly presents with a relapsing and remitting pattern. It affects the sensory nervous system causing neuropathic pain and paraesthesia, and can also affect the autonomic nervous system causing incontinence, urinary retention and erectile dysfunction.

Myasthenia gravis is a chronic neuromuscular disease caused by antibodies that disrupt the acetylcholine receptors in the neuromuscular junction. It presents with gradual onset weakness and starts by affecting the the extra-ocular muscles causing a complex ophthalmoplegia, and then moves downwards to affect the proximal muscles. It wouldn't cause fasciculations and doesn't affect the deep tendon reflexes or sensory nervous system.

10. E
Hypotension

L-3,4-dihydroxyphenylalanine (L-DOPA) is a precursor to dopamine and is converted to dopamine by L-DOPA decarboxylase. The idea behind using L-DOPA in the treatment of Parkinson's disease is that it can replace the lack of dopamine. However it can also cause side effects. These can be split into central and peripheral side effects. Central side effects include dyskinesia, hallucinations, insomnia and vivid dreams. These are caused by conversion of L-DOPA into dopamine in the brain. Peripheral side effects include nausea, vomiting and hypotension, and occur due to peripheral conversion.

Carbidopa is an L-DOPA decarboxylase inhibitor, which doesn't cross the blood brain barrier. Therefore it is used to prevent peripheral side effects of L-DOPA. If L-DOPA is converted to dopamine in the peripheries it can displace noradrenaline at the alpha 1 and 2 receptors on blood vessels. This prevents noradrenaline activity and can cause hypotension. Carbidopa acts to prevent this.

11. E
Meningioma of the falx cerbri

Meningiomas can occur in elderly patients and are often asymptomatic. They classically occur along the falx cerbri. Therefore they can cause bilateral leg weakness, by compressing both frontal lobes, whereas most brain tumours cause unilateral symptoms. They can eventually lead to raised intracranial pressure and seizures, and they also have a strong association with neurofibromatosis type 2.

Gliobastoma multiforme is the most aggressive primary brain tumour and commonly causes personality changes due to it affecting the frontal and temporal lobes. If it were present in the left frontal lobe, it would cause right-sided weakness and upper motor neurone signs.

Anterior spinal artery syndrome is also known as anterior spinal cord syndrome and is caused by ischaemia of the anterior spinal artery, resulting in loss of function of the anterior two-thirds of the spinal cord. This causes motor paralysis due to interruption of the corticospinal tracts, and loss of pain and temperature sensation due to interruption of the spinothalamic tracts, below the level of the lesion.

Multiple sclerosis is caused by demyelination of the central nervous system and leads to a mixture of motor and sensory signs. It would be very unlikely to occur in an elderly patient and is more common in younger patients, between 20-50 years old. Neither multiple sclerosis or anterior spinal artery syndrome would present with a headache.

Chronic inflammatory demyelinating polyneuropathy (CIDP) is an acquired immune-mediated inflammatory disorder of the peripheral nervous system, which also presents with both sensory and lower motor neurone signs. Therefore it would present with downward going plantars and also wouldn't cause a headache.

12. E
Epilepsy

This patient has had a seizure and subsequently developed a Todd's palsy. A Todd's palsy is where following a seizure there is transient weakness, and the patient's speech can also be affected. These symptoms often resolve within 24 hours. The reason eplilepsy the most likely diagnosis is because of her age, and the fact she was tired and confused upon waking.

A transient ischaemic attack (TIA) and ischaemic stroke would be very unlikely in a patient of this age. Also an ischaemic stroke would be the incorrect diagnosis in this case because her symptoms resolved within 24 hours.

A migrane could lead to weakness, and tiredness but is less likely to cause complete loss of consciousness.

Multiple sclerosis has a relapsing and remitting pattern. The symptoms of a relapse often take a few days to disappear and a full recovery after 12 hours is very unlikely.

13. D
Posterior communicating artery aneurysm

This patient has what is known as a 'surgical third nerve palsy'. This is where a posterior communicating artery aneurysm is compressing the outer part of the oculomotor nerve. The parasympathetic supply to the eye is carried on the outside of the nerve so this is affected as well as the motor function.

Diabetic neuropathy can also cause a third nerve palsy, but this causes pupil sparing, where the pupil is still reactive to light.

Horner's syndrome is caused by damage to the sympathetic chain. It presents with ptosis, miosis, anhidrosis and enophthalmos.

Argyll Robertson pupil is caused by damage to the parasympathetic pathways supplying the iris. The pupil is constricted and unreactive to light but can react to accommodation. It occurs in neurosyphilis and diabetes mellitus.

A lacunar infarction would cause symptoms affecting the whole of one side of the body. It wouldn't just affect the eye.

14. D
Right midbrain

This patient has Weber's syndrome, which is caused by a midbrain infarct. It causes an ipsilateral oculomotor nerve palsy and a contralateral hemiparesis. It has affected the right side, causing a right sided oculomotor nerve palsy and left sided hemiparesis.

A lateral medullary infarct would cause Wallenberg syndrome (ispilateral loss of pain and temperature on the face and contralateral loss on the torso). An infarct of the posterior limb of the internal capsule would cause a complete contralateral hemiparesis, with no sensory loss.

A basilar artery infarct presents with sudden neurological impairment, often loss of consciousness or even sudden death. If at the top of the artery it causes visual and oculomotor deficits, with normal motor function. If the infarct is at the mid portion it can cause 'locked in' syndrome, which is a complete loss of movement with preserved consciousness.

A left middle cerebral artery infarct would cause right sided weakness affecting the face and the torso. The leg is less likely to be effected. There would be sparing of the forehead, and also sensation would be affected. If the left hemisphere is dominant, then an infarct may cause Broca's expressive dysphasia and Wernicke's receptive dysphasia.

15. D
Friedreich's ataxia

Friedreich's ataxia is an autosomal recessive condition caused by expansions in a trinucleotide repeat within the frataxin gene. It causes degeneration of the spinocerebellar tracts (causing ataxia, nystagmus and dysarthria), degeneration of the corticospinal tracts (causing weakness and upward going plantars), dorsal column degeneration (causing loss of vibration, proprioception and deep tendon reflexes) and peripheral nerve damage. This condition is also associated with kyphoscoliosis, pes cavus, diabetes mellitus and hypertrophic obstructive cardiomyopathy (HOCM). This patient has also developed HOCM, which would explain his recurrent syncopal episodes.

Other causes of absent knee, and ankle reflexes, with upward going planters include amyotrophic lateral sclerosis, subacute combined degeneration of the spinal cord and tabes dorsalis (which occurs in neurosyphilis).

Congenital syphilis infection would present soon after birth with Hutchinson's triad (deafness, keratitis and sharp teeth).

Subacute combined degeneration of the spinal cord occurs as a result of vitamin B12 deficiency. It causes loss of the dorsal columns and corticospinal tracts. It can cause ataxia due to a loss of proprioception, but wouldn't cause nystagmus or dysarthria, as there is no cerebellar involvement.

Neuromyelitis optica, otherwise known as Devic's syndrome would present with optic neuritis and transverse myelitis.

Ataxic telangiectasia is an autosomal recessive condition, which comprises of cerebellar degeneration and multiple telangiectasia. These patients also have recurrent infections due to a weak immune system.

16. A
α-synuclein

This patient has developed Lewy body dementia (LBD), which presents with hallucinations and fluctuation of cognition. Patients later develop Parkinsonism. The same pathological process as idiopathic Parkinson's disease causes LBD. It is due to the deposition of α-synuclein (which forms Lewy bodies) in areas of the brain. In Parkinson's disease the deposition occurs in the substantia nigra of the midbrain.

β-amyloid and tau are found in Alzheimer's disease.

TDP-43 is associated with acquired amyotrophic lateral sclerosis and frontotemporal dementia. (Tau can also be found in frontotemporal dementia.)

SOD1 is associated with inherited amyotrophic lateral sclerosis.

17. B
Frontotemporal dementia

Frontotemporal dementia and amyotrophic lateral sclerosis are very strongly linked. Many patients who develop one of the conditions are likely to develop the other. Frontotemporal dementia presents with symptoms of disinhibition and personality changes due to frontal lobe involvement. If the left temporal lobe is involved it can cause semantic dementia, which is the loss of understanding the meanings of words, and difficulty word finding.

Alzheimer's disease is another form of dementia. It begins with a gradual loss of memory and spatial disorientation, which means patients get lost easily or forget where they have put things. As it progresses over many years there is personality change, with patients becoming more agitated. There is a loss of executive function. Finally there is global cognitive impairment and patients enter a neurovegetative state.

Depression is characterised by low mood, fatigue and anhedonia. It can lead to what is known as a pseudodementia. This presents with a more rapid onset, patients often answer 'I don't know' to questions, and may become distressed when asked questions that they don't know the answers to. It is also fully reversible. In true dementia patients often get questions wrong and can be quite apathetic about it.

Delirium has a rapid onset and is characterised by the following: disordered thinking, labile mood, impaired speech, hallucinations, and reversal of the sleep wake cycle, inattention and disorientation.

Riluzole acts by blocking TTX-sensitive sodium channels and is used to treat amyotrophic lateral sclerosis. Its side effects include nausea, weakness, headaches and rarely interstitial lung disease. It is thought to increase survival by 2–3 months.

18. A
Carbamazepine

Carbamazepine is used mainly to treat partial seizures. It is a P450 enzyme inducer. Inducers take a few weeks to take effect. During this time the patient's levels of carbamazepine remained stable. However once the P450 inducer effect took place it meant that carbamazepine metabolism by the liver was increased and thus the plasma levels decreased. This left the patient more susceptible to having seizures.

Sodium valproate is a P450 enzyme inhibitor and the other drugs listed do not affect the P450 system.

19. D
Pellegra

Pellegra is caused by nicotinic acid deficiency. It presents with a classic triad of dementia, diarrhoea and dermatitis (Casal's necklace is an erythematous rash that occurs in dermatomes C3 and C4). It can also cause insomnia, depression, neuropathy and seizures. Its causes include use of isoniazid and carcinoid syndrome.

Whipple's disease is caused by Tropheryma whipplei and presents with arthralgia, gastrointestinal symptoms (diarrhoea, weight loss, abdominal pain and malabsorption) and neurological symptoms (reversible dementia, ophthalmopelgia and facial myoclonus).

Toxoplasmosis occurs in immunocompromised individuals. It causes a posterior uveitis and encephalitis, which can present with seizures and focal neurological signs.

Neurosyphilis occurs after a prolonged syphilis infection. It causes tabes dorsalis, which is the degeneration of the dorsal columns and general paresis of the insane, which presents as dementia and psychosis.

Thiamine deficiency starts by causing Wernicke's encephalopathy. This is a reversible condition that presents with an ophthalmoplegia, ataxia and confusion. If not treated this can progress to Korsakoff's syndrome, which is an irreversible form of dementia caused by degeneration of the mammillary bodies. It is characterised by the inability to form new memories and confabulation.

20. D
Amitriptyline

This patient is suffering from recurrent migranes. These are classically unilateral throbbing headaches that are preceded by a visual aura and accompanied by nausea, vomiting, photophobia and phonophobia. If a patient is having two or more per month, they should be started on some form of prophylaxis. The first line treatment is propranolol, however this patient is asthmatic and therefore beta-blockers are contraindicated.

Other potential prophylactic agents include topiramate and amitriptyline. Topiramate is teratogenic; therefore the most appropriate drug would be amitriptyline. Sumatriptan, paracetamol and metoclopramide are drugs that can all be used in the acute setting, but not as prophylaxis.

21. C
Magnetic resonance imaging (MRI) scan of the head

This patient has new onset unilateral sensorineural deafness. The first diagnosis that needs to be ruled out is a tumour of the cerebellopontine angle, such as an acoustic neuroma. These tumours present with damage to the trigeminal nerve causing a loss of sensation on the face, a facial nerve palsy and sensorineural deafness.

Audiometry would help confirm the nature of the deafness, but we already know it is sensorineural. Otoscopy would give a view of the tympanic membrane and would be the first investigation if this patient had conductive hearing loss. Facial nerve electromyography is used to record electrical activity in the facial muscles. Nerve conduction studies can be used in Bell's palsy to predict recovery times. The facial nerve can be affected in a cerebellopontine angle tumours and therefore the nerve conduction is likely to be affected, but nerve conduction studies wouldn't confirm the underlying cause.

Serum calcium, phosphate and ALP tests can be ordered if patients are suspected to have Paget's disease. It would cause normal calcium, normal phosphate and raised ALP. This is a condition that leads to increased bone turnover and bone remodelling. It can cause sensorineural deafness due to remodelling of the petrosal bone, leading to compression of the vestibulo-cochlear nerve. It would also cause deep boring bone pain, and other complications include pathological fractures, osteosarcoma, high output congestive cardiac failure, and hypercalcaemia if patients are immobile.

22. D
Electrocardiogram (ECG)

Donepezil is an acetylcholinesterase inhibitor, which is used to treat Alzheimer's disease. It acts to increase the levels of acetylcholine in the brain, which are depleted in Alzheimer's disease. It is contraindicated in patients with cardiac conduction abnormalities, as it can worsen heart block. Therefore patients must be screened with an ECG. It is also contraindicated in patients with previous history of peptic ulcers, asthma and chronic obstructive pulmonary disease (COPD). Side effects include nausea, vomiting, diarrhoea, incontinence and insomnia.

23. D
Otoscopy

This patient has developed a lower motor neurone facial nerve palsy, which presents with unilateral weakness of the facial muscles. An upper motor neurone lesion would cause sparing of the forehead, so patients would be able to raise their eyebrows. The most common cause of lower motor neurone facial nerve palsy is an idiopathic Bell's palsy. But before this diagnosis can be made, other causes must be ruled out. Another common cause is Ramsay Hunt syndrome. This is caused by reactivation of a latent varicella zoster virus within the geniculate ganglion of the facial nerve. It causes a painful vesicular rash within the auditory canal. Therefore otoscopy should be carried out to look for these vesicles; and if seen aciclovir should be added to the treatment. Lyme disease serology may also be requested.

A computed tomography (CT) scan of the head would be requested if this were caused by an upper motor neurone lesion to look for any evidence of ischaemia or a space occupying lesion.

A facial nerve EMG may be used once the diagnosis is confirmed to predict the length of recovery, but it wouldn't influence the treatment.

Testing visual acuity isn't required in this patient, but she would require good eye care if she is unable to close her eye completely. This involves use of an eye patch and lubricants.

Audiometry is also not required, as this condition doesn't affect the patient's hearing. It can cause paralysis of the stapedius muscle, leading to hyperacusis, but this can be diagnosed from the history and on examination.

24. D
Lead poisoning

Lead poisoning presents with a peripheral neuropathy that primarily affects the lower limbs. Other signs include memory loss, depression, insomnia, joint pains and fatigue. On examination a blue tinge can be seen on the patient's gums, and X-rays may show dense metaphyseal lines. Complications include anaemia and renal failure.

Chronic inflammatory demyelinating polyneuropathy (CIDP) is an autoimmune condition affecting the peripheral nerves, and mainly affecting the motor neurones. On examination lower motor neurone signs such as fasciculations, atrophy, weakness and hyporeflexia can be seen.

Vitamin B12 deficiency can lead to subacute combined degeneration of the spinal cord, which can present with ataxia, loss of knee and ankle reflexes, and upward going plantars. There may also be a sensory peripheral neuropathy, signs of anaemia and glossitis.

Chemotherapy agents such as vincristine and cisplatin are known to cause a peripheral neuropathy. However this is mainly a sensory neuropathy and doesn't usually affect the motor neurones, so they would be unlikely to cause weakness.

Acute intermittent porphyria is an autosomal dominant condition that can result in a build up of porphyrins due to the lack of the porphobilinogen deaminase gene. It presents with a crisis that affects multiple systems in the body. Gastrointestinal symptoms include abdominal pain, vomiting and constipation. Neuropsychiatric symptoms include psychosis, peripheral neuropathy and seizures due to hyponatraemia. Cardiovascular symptoms include hypertension and tachycardia.

25. D
Posterior limb of the internal capsule

The posterior limb of the internal capsule is where the motor fibres arising from the motor cortex of the brain travel through before forming the corticospinal tracts; and its blood supply arises from the lenticulostriate branches of the middle cerebral artery. This is a small area that contains a high concentration of motor fibres. An infarct here causes a complete contralateral hemiparesis without sensory deficit.

The ventral posterolateral nucleus of the thalamus lies within the internal capsule, and an infarct here would lead to a complete contralateral sensory loss.

The anterior cerebral artery infarcts mainly affect the lower limbs, while middle cerebral artery infarcts affect the face, torso and upper limbs, and both would cause motor and sensory symptoms.

Posterior cerebral artery infarcts affect the visual fields causing a contralateral homonymous hemianopia with macular sparing.

26. A
Posterior inferior cerebellar artery

This patient has developed Wallenberg syndrome (lateral medullary syndrome) due to an infarction of the posterior inferior cerebellar artery, which presents with ipsilateral loss of pain and temperature sensation on the face, and contralateral loss on the torso. It can cause ipsilateral Horner's syndrome (which is described above as partial ptosis, miosis, and anhidrosis). Other signs include dysarthria (due to its effect on cranial nerves IX and X), nystagmus and vertigo (due to its effect on the vestibular nucleus) and ataxia (due to its effect on the inferior cerebellar peduncle).

A basilar artery infarct presents with sudden neurological impairment, often loss of consciousness or even sudden death. If at the top of the artery it causes visual and oculomotor deficits, with normal motor function. If the infarct is at the mid portion it can cause 'locked in' syndrome, which is a complete loss of movement with preserved consciousness.

Middle cerebral artery infarcts affect the face, torso and upper limbs causing a mixture of motor and sensory symptoms. The lenticulostriate arteries supply the internal capsule and an infarct here is called a lacunar infarct. These infarcts can be pure motor, pure sensory or mixed. They affect the whole of one side of the body and don't cause any cerebellar signs.

An anterior spinal artery infarct causes what is known as anterior spinal syndrome. The anterior spinal artery supplies blood to the anterior two thirds of the spinal cord. If the blood flow is interrupted it causes complete motor paralysis and loss of pain and temperature sensation below the level of the infarct. Vibration and proprioception remain intact.

27. D
Otoscopy revealed evidence of blood in the middle ear

Blood in the middle ear is also known as haemotypanum, and is a sign of a basilar skull fracture. Other signs indicating a basilar skull fracture are racoon eyes, Battle's sign, and cerebrospinal fluid (CSF) leakage from the nose or ears. If any of these signs are present they warrant an urgent CT scan of the head.

Other criteria for performing a CT scan of the head following a head injury are a GCS of less than 13 on initial assessment, a GCS of less than 15 following 2 hours in the accident and emergency (A&E) department, suspected open or depressed skull fracture, focal neurological deficit, post traumatic seizure, more than one episode of vomiting or anticoagulation. (Aspirin and clopidogrel are antiplatelet drugs; anticoagulation refers to drugs such as warfarin.) Tongue biting can be a sign of seizure activity, however if it occurs during a seizure it classically affects the side of the tongue. This patient didn't lose consciousness at any point making a seizure an unlikely cause of the fall, and no post fall seizure activity has been described.

28. B
Betahistine

This patient has developed Meniere's disease, which presents with vertigo, tinnitus and sensorineural deafness. Betahistine is a histamine H3-receptor antagonist and can be used as prophylaxis against attacks. In severe cases endolymphatic surgery is required.

Both prochlorperazine and cinnarizine can be used in the acute setting. They are both antiemetics that are good at treating vertigo. Prochlorperazine is a dopamine D2-receptor antagonist, and cinnarizine is an antihistamine which binds to the H1-receptors.

Metoclopramide is an antiemetic and pro-kinetic drug, which also acts as a dopamine D2-receptor antagonist but has no role in treating Meniere's disease.

The Epley manoeuver is used in benign positional vertigo to clear debris from the semicircular canals that make up the vestibular apparatus.

29. C
Subdural haemorrhage

This is a haemorrhage occurring between the dura and arachnoid layers of the meninges. It occurs due to rupture of the bridging veins. Risk factors are anything that causes brain atrophy (such as dementia and alcoholism), which leads to increased tension on the bridging veins. Recurrent falls is also a risk factor. Subdural haemorrhages can present very insidiously often with fluctuating consciousness, sleepiness, headache and personality change.

Alzheimer's disease is a cause of dementia and is common in the elderly, but would progress at a much slower rate.

Vascular dementia is caused by recurrent ischaemic strokes, and presents with a stepwise progression. This patient doesn't have any vascular risk factors and doesn't have any focal neurology.

Depression is cause of pseudo-dementia and therefore is reversible. This patient would be at risk of depression especially because of his alcohol history and age. However it wouldn't explain his rapid decline in cognitive function.

Korsakoff's syndrome is an irreversible form of dementia that occurs in alcoholics as a result of chronic thiamine deficiency. It causes degeneration of the mammillary bodies and would present with confabulation.

30. B
Isotretinoin

This lady his developed idiopathic intracranial hypertension, which typically occurs in obese females, and presents with headache, blurred vision, bilateral abducens nerve palsy, and papillodema. Its cause is often unknown but it can be due to use of the following drugs: isotretinoin, vitamin A, tetracyclines, nitrofurantoin, oral contraceptives, and growth hormone. Isotretinion is a retinoid, which is used to treat severe acne. Its other side effects include dryness of the skin, eyes and mouth, hepatitis, hypercholestrolaemia, depression and teratogenicity.

GTN spray and nifedipine (a calcium channel blocker) can both cause a headache as a result of vasodilation.

Codeine phosphate is a weak opiate and can cause an analgesic headache if it is used too much. Other analgesic drugs such as paracetamol and non-steroidal anti-inflammatory drugs (NSAIDs) can also cause an analgesic headache, but codeine phosphate is one of the worst culprits.

Caffeine is a stimulant and can result in a headache if it is rapidly withdrawn after prolonged use.

Renal and Urology Questions

1. A 35-year-old male presents to his doctor with a fever and backache. He also complains of a poor stream when urinating. A rectal examination reveals a regularly enlarged but tender and boggy prostate. Which of the following drugs should this patient be prescribed?

A. Amoxicillin
B. Trimethoprim
C. Ciprofloxacin
D. Doxazosin
E. Finasteride

2. A patient presents to hospital with severe colicky flank pain, which radiates from her flank to her groin. She has vomited twice and feels nauseous. For a few days prior to this she experienced dysuria, urinary frequency and urgency. Her urine dipstick shows haematuria, raised leucocytes and nitrites. A computed tomography scan of the kidneys, ureters and bladder (CT KUB) shows a staghorn calculus present in the left renal pelvis. Which of the following bacteria is most likely to be causing this patient's symptoms?

A. Escherichia coli
B. Enterococcus faecalis
C. Staphylococcus saprophyticus
D. Proteus mirabilis
E. Serratia marcescens

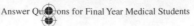
3. A 20-year-old man known to have nephrotic syndrome presents to hospital with sudden onset severe left flank pain. On examination his left kidney is enlarged. His blood tests show a rise in his serum creatinine and his urine dip shows haematuria and proteinuria. Which of the following is the most likely underlying diagnosis?

A. Pyelonephritis
B. Renal calculus
C. Renal cyst rupture
D. Renal vein thrombosis
E. Splenic rupture

4. A patient known to have a human immunodeficiency virus (HIV) infection presents to hospital with pitting oedema. He also describes his urine as being frothy. A urine dip on admission shows proteinuria, but no haematuria. A renal biopsy is taken and shows deposition of IgM and C3 in some of the glomeruli. What is the most likely underlying diagnosis?

A. Mesangiocapillary glomerulonephritis type II
B. IgA nephropathy
C. Proliferative glomerulonephritis
D. Anti-glomerular basement membrane disease
E. Focal segmental glomerulosclerosis

5. A 34-year-old woman was prescribed captopril to treat her hypertension. Two weeks later a blood test was performed and showed her serum creatinine levels had doubled. As part of the investigations a renal angiogram is carried out and shows the renal arteries having a string of beads appearance. Which of the following should be used to treat this patient's hypertension?

A. Prednisolone and cyclophosphamide
B. Lamivudine and interferon alpha
C. Amlodipine
D. Losartan
E. Percutaneous balloon angioplasty

6. A 22-year-old male, with a diagnosis of Alport's syndrome, presents to his doctor with persistent haematuria. He goes on to develop chronic renal failure, and as a result receives a renal transplant. A few months after the transplant he develops severe haematuria, proteinuria and hypertension. Which of the following would you expect to see on a renal biopsy?

A. Normal renal biopsy
B. Anti-glomerular basement membrane antibodies
C. IgA and C3 deposited in the glomerulus
D. Tramline appearance of a double basement membrane
E. Fusion of the podocytes seen on electron microscopy

7. A 35-year-old woman presents to hospital with a fever and oliguria. Whilst in hospital her conscious level decreases and five minutes later she has a seizure. On examination she is found to be jaundiced and also have bilateral pitting oedema. Her blood tests and urine dipstick show the following:

Haemoglobin: 71 g/L
White cell count: 10.1×10^9/L
Platelet count: 56×10^9/L
Blood film: Schistocytes
Urinary haemoglobin: ++
Urinary protein: +++

Which of the following is the most likely diagnosis?

A. Paroxysmal nocturnal haemoglobinuria
B. Disseminated intravascular coagulation
C. Pre-eclampsia
D. Haemolytic uraemic syndrome
E. Thrombotic thrombocytopenic purpura

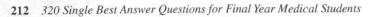

8. A patient with stage 5 chronic kidney disease presents to hospital with sharp central chest pain. The pain is worse on inspiration and when he lies down. The pain can be relieved slightly by sitting forwards. Which of the following treatment regimes should be started to treat this patient's underlying condition?

A. Primary coronary angioplasty
B. Haemodialysis
C. Colchicine
D. Diclofenac
E. Allopurinol

9. A 65-year-old patient presents with lower back pain. A magnetic resonance imaging (MRI) scan is requested and this patient is found to have lytic lesions in his lumbar spine. Serum electrophoresis shows a monoclonal protein band. Which of the following is most likely to be found when analysing this patient's urine?

A. Low calcium
B. Bence-Jones proteins
C. Plasma cells
D. Myoglobinuria
E. Raised nitrites

10. A patient with poorly controlled type 2 diabetes mellitus and end stage renal failure attends his local hospital for a routine dialysis session. During his dialysis session he develops sudden onset crushing central chest pain and vomits once. Which of the following is the most likely underlying diagnosis?

A. Pulmonary embolism
B. Pericarditis
C. Myocarditis
D. Myocardial infarction
E. Oesophageal spasm

11. A patient with a known history of polycystic kidney disease presents to hospital with a sudden onset severe headache and neck stiffness. Which of the following is the most likely underlying diagnosis?

A. Subarachnoid haemorrhage
B. Meningitis
C. Venous sinus thrombosis
D. Migraine
E. Hypertensive encephalopathy

12. An elderly patient who is on haemodialyisis for chronic renal failure has deteriorated recently. He decides he no longer wants to be treated with haemodialysis and he has full capacity to make this decision. Haemodialysis is withdrawn from his treatment. Following this he develops myoclonic jerks. Which of the following medications should he be prescribed to control his new symptoms?

A. Haloperidol
B. Clonazepam
C. Sodium bicarbonate
D. Lanthanum carbonate
E. Alfacalcidol

13. A patient who was prescribed high dose benzylpenicillin to treat a Streptococcal infection develops oliguria. He also develops a fever, rash and arthralgia. His blood tests show an eosinophilia and a renal biopsy shows infiltration of the renal interstitium with T-lymphocytes and macrophages. Which of the following is the most likely cause of his acute kidney injury?

A. Acute tubular necrosis
B. Proliferative glomerulonephritis
C. Tubulointerstitial nephritis
D. Sepsis
E. Obstructive uropathy

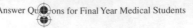

14. A patient presents to his doctor with haematuria two weeks after an erysipelas skin infection. He is oliguric and his blood pressure is 160/90 mmHg (normally it is 120/80 mmHg). A urine dipstick shows both haematuria and proteinuria. A renal biopsy is performed. Which of the following is most likely to be found in the glomeruli?

A. IgA and C3 deposition
B. IgM and C3 deposition
C. IgG and C3 deposition
D. IgA and C4 deposition
E. IgG and C4 deposition

15. A patient suffering from severe open angle glaucoma is prescribed acetazolamide. Which of the following is a side effect of acetazolamide?

A. Renal tubular acidosis type 1
B. Renal tubular acidosis type 2
C. Renal tubular acidosis type 4
D. Hypernatraemia
E. Hyperkalaemia

16. A patient with a history of renal stones presents with renal colic. A computed tomography scan of the kidneys, ureters and bladder (CT KUB) is performed but the renal stone cannot be seen. Following ureteroscopy a 5 mm renal calculus is removed. Which of the following medications is likely to be responsible for the formation of this stone?

A. Furosemide
B. Acetazolamide
C. Alfacalcidol
D. Indinavir sulphate
E. Senna

17. A 40-year-old male presents to hospital with colicky abdominal pain in his left flank, which radiates down to his groin. On further questioning he states he is nauseated and has vomited three times on the way to hospital. He is currently experiencing dysuria. Which of the following should be given in hospital as a form of analgesia?

A. Oral naproxen
B. Diclofenac suppository
C. Intravenous paracetamol
D. Intravenous morphine
E. Oral co-codamol

18. A 60-year-old male presents with visible painless haematuria. He undergoes investigation and is diagnosed with a squamous cell carcinoma of the bladder. Which of the following is the greatest risk factor for developing squamous cell carcinoma of the bladder?

A. Age
B. Working with aromatic amines
C. Pelvic radiation
D. Schistosomiasis
E. Treatment with cyclophosphamide

19. A 35-year-old female with no significant past medical history has recently developed urinary incontinence. She states that she has a sudden urge to pass urine, almost immediately followed by complete uncontrolled emptying of the bladder. She denies having haematuria, vaginal bleeding or dyspareunia. Which of the following treatments is most likely to help relieve this patient's symptoms?

A. Tolterodine
B. Duloxetine
C. Doxazosin
D. Burch colposuspension
E. Topical oestriol cream

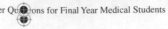

20. A 21-year-old male presents to his doctor with a painless lump on his left testicle. On examination the lump is hard and non-tender. It doesn't transluminate. Which of the following is the most likely underlying diagnosis?

A. Haematocele
B. Varicocele
C. Hydrocele
D. Teratoma
E. Seminoma

21. A patient with autosomal dominant polycystic kidney disease has reached end stage renal failure, and is about to undergo his first dialysis session. Routine blood tests are taken. Which of the following is most likely to be within the normal range in this patient?

A. Haemoglobin
B. Serum phosphate
C. Serum urate
D. Serum creatinine
E. Parathyroid hormone

22. A patient with ongoing membranous nephropathy has developed hypoalbuminaemia, as a result of proteinuria. Which of the following drugs would reduce the loss of albumin via the kidneys?

A. Amiloride
B. Bumetanide
C. Candesartan
D. Indapamide
E. Human albumin solution

23. An 85-year-old man presents with nocturia. On taking a full history he reveals that recently he has had increased urinary frequency, hesitancy and terminal dribbling when passing urine. On systems review he states he has been suffering from a dull backache and lost 5 kg in the last month. Which of the following investigations should be used to confirm the underlying diagnosis?

A. Cystoscopy
B. Transrectal ultrasound and biopsy of the prostate
C. Prostate specific antigen levels
D. Serum calcium, phosphate and alkaline phosphatase (ALP) levels
E. Magnetic resonance imaging (MRI) scan of the prostate

24. A 75-year-old lady with a history of rheumatoid arthritis is found to have hypoalbuminaemia during a routine blood test. Subsequent investigation with a urine dip reveals proteinuria. Her renal biopsy showed a diffusely thickened basement membrane. Which of the following drugs has she been prescribed that may be responsible for her proteinuria?

A. Methotrexate
B. Sulfasalazine
C. Naproxen
D. Penicillamine
E. Leflunomide

25. A 22-year-old epileptic male is brought into hospital following a prolonged 40-minute tonic clonic seizure. He is eventually sedated and intubated by an anaesthetist. His seizure is under control. In the intensive care unit he is catheterised and it is noticed that his urine is a dark brown colour. Which of the following treatments should be initiated immediately?

A. Intravenous dexamethasone
B. 1 litre of 0.9% saline STAT
C. Intravenous insulin and 50% dextrose
D. Intravenous sodium bicarbonate
E. Haemodialysis

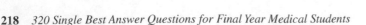
26. An overdose of which of the following medications can be treated with haemodialysis?

A. Aspirin
B. Paracetamol
C. Amitriptyline
D. Diazepam
E. Propranolol

27. A 32-year-old lady is currently on an immunosuppressive regime following a renal transplant. She attends her nephrologist for a follow-up appointment where she receives the results of her routine blood tests. She is told that her fasting venous glucose and HbA1c are both raised. Which of the following drugs is most likely to be responsible for this?

A. Mercaptopurine
B. Mycophenolate motefil
C. Cyclophosphamide
D. Tacrolimus
E. Basiliximab

28. A 35-year-old male presents to hospital with dyspnea, cough and haemoptysis. He also reports haematuria. His urine dipstick shows haematuria and proteinuria. His initial blood tests show a raised white cell count (differential showing an eosinophilia), raised serum urea, erythrocyte sedimentation rate (ESR), C-reactive protein (CRP) and perinuclear anti-neutrophil cytoplasmic antibodies (P-ANCA). Which of the following is the most likely underlying diagnosis?

A. Granulomatosis with polyangiitis
B. Microscopic polyangiitis
C. Eosinophilic granulomatosis with polyangiitis
D. Anti-glomerular basement membrane disease
E. Kawasaki disease

29. A 52-year-old male is started on ramipril by his doctor to treat his high blood pressure. Three days later he presented to hospital with a cough, dyspnea, and wheeze, which is made worse by lying down. On examination he was found to have bilateral fine inspiratory crackles throughout both lungs. His arterial blood gas showed a type 1 respiratory failure. Which of the following conditions is this patient likely to have, which has resulted in his symptoms?

A. Acquired angioedema
B. Asthma
C. Bilateral renal artery stenosis
D. Acute urinary obstruction
E. Congestive cardiac failure

30. A 70-year-old man is referred to a nephrologist for worsening kidney function. His doctor noticed a gradual rise in his creatinine over the past few years. On examination the nephrologist found two large ballotable masses, one in each flank and a non-tender suprapubic mass, which is dull to percussion. A rectal examination revealed an enlarged prostate. Which of the following is the most likely cause of his decline in renal function?

A. Amyloidosis
B. Polycystic kidney disease
C. Hydronephrosis
D. Bilateral renal artery stenosis
E. Metastatic lung cancer

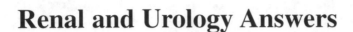

Renal and Urology Answers

1. C
Ciprofloxacin

This patient has prostatitis. This presents with a fever, back pain, urinary symptoms (dysuria, frequency and haematuria), haematospermia and a swollen prostate. Ciprofloxacin is a quinolone antibiotic and used because it is able to penetrate the prostate well.

Amoxicillin is used to treat urinary tract infections (UTIs) in pregnancy. Trimethoprim is used to treat UTIs in women who are not pregnant.

Doxazosin is an alpha-blocker, which can be used to treat benign prostatic hyperplasia, and to help expulsion of renal stones. It does so by causing relaxation of the smooth muscle in the ureters. It is also a third line antihypertensive drug.

Finasteride is a 5α-reductase inhibitor also used in benign prostatic hyperplasia. It inhibits the conversion of testosterone to the more potent dihydrotestosterone.

2. D
Proteus mirabilis

This patient has developed a kidney stone as a result of a urinary tract infection (UTI). The symptoms consistent with a renal stone are renal colic and pain radiating to the groin, nausea, vomiting and haematuria. Renal stones are a common cause of painful haematuria.

UTIs present with raised nitrites and leucocytes in the urine. Proteus mirabilis is a gram-negative anaerobe that can cause UTIs. It is also found in human faeces. It causes alkalinisation of the urine, by use of a urease enzyme, which converts urea to ammonia. This leads to formation of struvite stones (also known as magnesium ammonium phosphate stones). These are large radio-opaque stones and can form a staghorn calculus.

The other bacteria are all causes of UTIs, but are not associated with the development of renal stones. Escherichia coli is the most common cause of UTIs.

3. D
Renal vein thrombosis

This patient has developed a renal vein thrombus. Patients with nephrotic syndrome have a higher risk of renal vein thrombus development due to hypercoagulability caused by the loss of antithrombin III in the urine. Renal vein thrombosis would present with sudden onset flank pain, haematuria, a palpable kidney and a sudden deterioration in renal function. The mainstay of treatment is with anticoagulation and this could be initiated with low molecular weight heparin.

Pyelonephritis would also present with flank pain, but is also likely to cause dysuria and a fever, and the urine dip would be positive for leucocytes and nitrites. Pyelonephritis is common in young female patients but much less likely in male patients.

A renal calculus would present with flank pain radiating to the groin. The pain is often described as colicky and associated with nausea and vomiting. Renal calculi classically occur in patients 20-50 years old.

Renal cyst rupture can also present with sudden onset flank pain but would be more likely in a patient with underlying polycystic kidney disease.

Splenic rupture can occur following a history of blunt trauma to the abdomen. It would present with left upper quadrant abdominal pain and patients at risk include those with an Epstein-Barr virus (EBV) infection.

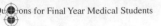

4. E
Focal segmental glomerulosclerosis

This patient has developed nephrotic syndrome as a result of focal segmental glomerulosclerosis. The frothy urine represents proteinuria and this patient also has oedema. The only feature missing from the nephrotic syndrome triad is hypoalbuminaemia. Focal segmental glomerulosclerosis is associated with HIV and heroin use, but can also be idiopathic. It presents with proteinuria or nephrotic syndrome and can progress to end stage renal failure. A renal biopsy would show that only parts of some glomeruli are affected, and would also show IgM and C3 deposition in the affected areas.

Mesangiocapillary glomerulonephritis type II is another cause of nephrotic syndrome, and occurs as a result of intramembranous deposits of C3. A renal biopsy shows mesangial proliferation and thickening of the capillary walls. This is described as a tramline appearance.

IgA nephropathy is otherwise known as Berger's disease and causes IgA deposition in the glomeruli. It causes a self-limiting haematuria, often following an acute viral infection.

Proliferative glomerulonephritis occurs a few weeks after a Streptococcal infection of the throat or skin. It normally presents with a nephritic picture (haematuria, proteinuria, raised blood pressure and renal impairment). The Streptococcal antigen gets deposited in the glomeruli and a renal biopsy shows IgG and C3 deposition around the mesangial and endothelial cells.

5. E
Percutaneous balloon angioplasty

This patient has fibromuscular dysplasia, which is an autosomal dominant disease, causing narrowing of the arteries in the kidneys, and also narrowing of the carotid arteries. It should be considered in young patients (especially females) who develop hypertension. It is diagnosed by use of a renal angiogram, which would show a string of beads appearance. Percutaneous balloon angioplasty is the first line treatment. In this case use of an angiotensin converting enzyme (ACE) inhibitor has caused dilation of the efferent arteriole in the glomeruli. Due to the blood supply already being compromised by the underlying condition, this causes a reduced pressure and reduced glomerular filtration rate (GFR), which has compromised renal function.

Prednisolone and cyclophosphamide is an immunosuppressive regime used to treat many of the glomerulonephritides (especially crescentic glomerulonephritis).

Lamivudine and interferon alpha is a combination of drugs used to treat hepatitis B. Hepatitis B is linked to polyarteritis nodosa, which is a medium vessel vasculitis that also affects the kidneys. However the renal angiogram shows aneurysms and thrombosis. These patients would also present with systemic signs and symptoms such as abdominal pain, fever, weight loss, mononeuritis multiplex, and livedo reticularis. They may also have signs of liver cirrhosis resulting from an underlying chronic hepatitis B infection.

Amlodipine is a dihydropyridine calcium channel blocker used to treat essential hypertension. This is the first line treatment of essential hypertension in Afro-Caribbean patients and patients over 55 years old. However in this case there is an underlying cause and therefore it should be treated.

Losartan is an angiotensin II receptor blocker, which can be used in patients that cannot tolerate an ACE inhibitor. However, like ACE inhibitors, it is contraindicated in this patient due to renal artery stenosis.

6. B
Anti-glomerular basement membrane antibodies

This patient has underlying Alport's syndrome. This disease has many forms but is most commonly inherited in an X-linked dominant pattern. It leads to a lack of collagen type IV in the basement membrane of the glomeruli. It presents with gradual bilateral sensorineural hearing loss, lenticonus and a gradual decline of renal function. It commonly causes persistent haematuria. It is treated with a renal transplant.

However, due to the transplant having collagen type IV in the glomerular basement membrane, the immune system sees this as a foreign antigen. As a result anti-glomerular basement membrane antibodies are produced. This presents with haematuria, oliguria and can cause rapidly progressive glomerulonephritis, which is diagnosed by use of a renal biopsy and immunofluorescence staining for IgG.

IgA and C3 deposits occur in both IgA nephropathy and Henoch-Schonlein purpura (HSP). IgA nephropathy (Berger's disease) is often self-limiting. HSP is a systemic form of IgA nephropathy. It is a small vessel ANCA negative vasculitis, which causes a purpuric rash on the extensor surfaces of the legs, polyarthritis and abdominal pain (due to gastrointestinal bleeding). It is more common in children than in adults.

Tramline appearance of a double basement membrane occurs in mesangiocapillary glomerulonephritis, which is due to thickened capillary walls and mesangial proliferation. It occurs as a result of either subendothelial (type1) or intramembranous (type 2) deposits.

Fusion of the podocytes occurs in minimal change glomerulonephritis. These changes cannot be seen under a light microscope and can only be seen by using an electron microscope. Minimal change glomerulonephritis is most common in children. It causes nephrotic syndrome and is associated with Hodgkin's lymphoma and non-steroidal anti-inflammatory drug (NSAID) use. It often responds well to steroids but patients are prone to relapse.

7. E
Thrombotic thrombocytopenic purpura

Thrombotic thrombocytopenic purpura presents with a fever, fluctuating neurological signs, microangiopathic haemolytic anaemia (resulting in schistocytes on the blood film, which is often severe enough to cause jaundice), thrombocytopenia, renal failure and haematuria and/or proteinuria. The cause is often unknown. There is a deficiency in ADAMTS13, which is a von Willebrand factor cleaving protease. As a result there are abnormally large von Willebrand factor mulitmers, which cause platelet

9"x6"
b3668_02-Endocrine.indd 37
b3668 320 Single Best Answer Questions for Final Year Medical Students
23-Aug-19 6

aggregation and fibrin deposition in small vessels. This is a medical emergency and requires plasma exchange, steroids, vincristine and immunoglobulins as part of the treatment regime.

Disseminated intravascular coagulation (DIC) would present with patients being unwell, having a purpuric rash and high risk of bleeding. It also causes microangiopathic haemolytic anaemia and low platelets but wouldn't present with the urinary signs.

Pre-eclampsia is a condition that can occur to women during pregnancy and it causes hypertension and proteinuria. It can progress to eclampsia (seizures).

Haemolytic uraemic syndrome (HUS) presents with a triad of microangiopathic haemolytic anaemia, thrombocytopenia and acute kidney injury. It is most commonly due to E. coli O157 and therefore patients can have a previous history of bloody diarrhoea. HUS occurs more commonly in children, and neurological symptoms are less likely.

Paroxysmal nocturnal haemoglobinuria is a rare condition that causes haemolysis (especially at night), marrow failure and also thrombophilia (leaving patients at risk of thromboembolism). As a result of intravascular haemolysis haemosiderin can be found in the urine. It doesn't cause shistocyte formation or renal impairment.

8. B
Haemodialysis

This patient has developed pericarditis as a result of uraemia. This is an indication for haemodialysis, which would reduce the levels of urea in the blood and therefore relieve this patient's symptoms.

Normally pericarditis would be treated with a non-steroidal anti-inflammatory drug (such as naproxen). The second line treatment is colchicine. However both of these drugs are contraindicated in severe renal failure. Also use of haemodialysis would be far more effective in uraemic pericarditis as it acts to remove the cause.

Allopurinol is a xanthine oxidase inhibitor and acts to reduce the production of uric acid. It is used to prevent gout and may also be used as long-term prophylaxis to prevent hyperuricaemia.

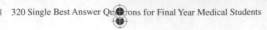

> Primary coronary angioplasty would be appropriate if this patient was having a myocardial infarction. Patients with renal failure are at a higher risk of myocardial infarctions, but this would present with central crushing chest pain, radiating to the jaw and left arm, and also cause sweating, nausea and vomiting.

9. B
Bence-Jones proteins

This patient has multiple myeloma. This is evident due to the lytic lesions found in the lumbar spine and also the presence of an M-band on serum electrophoresis (which represents a paraprotein). Multiple myeloma has detrimental effects on the kidneys. It causes hypercalcaemia, which results in nephrocalcinosis and renal stones. The high cell turnover leads to hyperuricaemia and this causes urate nephropathy. Bence-Jones proteins are part of the diagnostic criteria, and these are light immunoglobulin chains that are found in the urine. The kidneys are also affected by the deposition of AL-amyloid, which causes nephrotic syndrome.

Plasma cells are not found in the urine.

The urine has high calcium content due to hypercalcaemia.

Myoglobinuria occurs in rhabdomyolysis as a result of skeletal muscle cell breakdown and raised nitrites would occur in a urinary tract infection along with raised leucocytes.

10. D
Myocardial infarction

Patients with end stage renal failure are at a high risk of ischaemic heart disease. This patient also has a history of diabetes mellitus, which is another risk factor for ischaemic heart disease. The chest pain he is experiencing is consistent with a myocardial infarction.

A pulmonary embolism and pericarditis would present with pleuritic chest pain, and myocarditis and oesophageal spasm are more likely to present with a central crushing chest pain. However given the acute presentation, associated vomiting and cardiac risk factors, a myocardial infarction is the most likely underlying diagnosis.

11. A
Subarachnoid haemorrhage

Polycystic kidney disease is a genetic disorder in which the renal tubules become structurally abnormal, resulting in the development and growth of multiple cysts within the kidney. The most common form is autosomal dominant. Complications of this condition include renal cyst rupture, end stage renal failure, liver cysts, mitral valve prolapse and subarachnoid haemorrhage. Patients with polycystic kidney disease are at risk of developing intracranial berry aneurysms, which can rupture and cause a subarachnoid haemorrhage. The severity, acute onset and meninigitic features of the headache make this the most likely diagnosis.

Patients with polycystic kidney disease are also at risk of hypertension due to activation of the renin-angiotensin system. However there is no history of hypertension in this case and therefore hypertensive encephalopathy is less likely. In patients with polycystic kidney disease, hypertension is best treated by use of an angiotensin converting enzyme (ACE) inhibitor.

Meningitis would present with features of meningism such as neck stiffness, photophobia and phonophobia, and a fever.

A migraine would present with a unilateral throbbing headache and may be preceded by visual aura.

A venous sinus thrombosis can present with a headache, focal neurological signs and seizures. It would be more likely to occur in patients with underlying risk factors for thrombosis such as pregnancy, use of the combined oral contraceptive pill, underlying malignancy and antiphospholipid syndrome.

12. B
Clonazepam

Clonazepam is a benzodiazepine drug that is used to treat restless legs and myoclonic jerks in chronic kidney disease. Myoclonic jerks occur due to a build up of by-products in the body and present with twitches caused by sudden muscle contractions.

Haloperidol is a dopamine receptor antagonist and can be used to treat hallucinations that may occur once stopping dialysis.

Sodium bicarbonate can be given to counteract a metabolic acidosis that can occur in chronic kidney disease.

Lanthanum carbonate is a phosphate binder used to treat hyperphosphataemia. This presents with non-specific symptoms such as fatigue, anorexia, sleep disturbance, nausea and vomiting.

Alfacalcidol is a vitamin D supplement that is given in chronic kidney disease to treat vitamin D deficiency.

13. C
Tubulointerstitial nephritis

This patient has developed acute tubulointerstitial nephritis secondary to the penicillin he was prescribed. Other drugs that can cause this are cephalosporins, non-steroidal anti-inflammatory drugs, sulphonamides, omeprazole, thiazide and loop diuretics. It presents with acute kidney injury, fever, rash and arthralgia. Investigations would show an eosinophilia, raised serum IgE and eosinophils could be seen in the urine.

Acute tubular necrosis is caused either by nephrotoxic agents such as gentamicin or by ischaemia that occurs as a result of the poor perfusion of the kidneys in pre-renal acute kidney injury. It is characterised by the death of the tubular epithelial cells and is diagnosed by the presence of 'muddy brown casts' of epithelial cells in the urine.

Proliferative glomerulonephritis can occur as a result of a Streptococcal infection, however often occurs a few weeks after the infection and the renal biopsy would show evidence of proliferation.

Sepsis is a cause of pre-renal acute kidney injury and the hypotension that occurs in sepsis leads to poor perfusion of the kidneys. This could have been the underlying cause in this patient, however the other features in the history make tubulointerstitial nephritis more likely.

An obstructive uropathy would present with oliguria and could be due to any condition that obstructs the ureters or urethra. Causes would include renal calculi, bladder cancer and prostate cancer.

14. C
IgG and C3 deposition

This patient has developed poststreptococcal glomerulonephritis. This is caused by Streptococcus pyogenes, which can either cause a skin infection or a Streptococcal sore throat (which can result in scarlet fever and rheumatic fever). A few weeks after the infection there may be deposition of immune complexes in the glomerulus, which can result in a type III hypersensitivity reaction. It presents with nephritic syndrome. Often if the history is clear, a renal biopsy is not required for diagnosis. However if it is carried out then it would show a proliferative glomerulonephritis with both IgG and C3 deposition in the glomeruli.

IgA and C3 deposition occurs in Berger's disease (IgA nephropathy), which presents with haematuria and is often self-limiting. It normally follows a viral infection. It can also be found in Henoch-Schonlein purpura (HSP), which is a more systemic form that presents with a purpuric rash on the extensor surfaces of the legs, abdominal pain and polyarthritis.

IgM and C3 deposition occurs in focal segmental glomerulosclerosis, which would normally present with nephrotic syndrome.

IgA and C4 deposition, and IgG and C4 deposition is not a classic finding in any of the glomerulonephritides.

15. B
Renal tubular acidosis type 2

Acetazolamide is a carbonic anhydrase inhibitor. Carbonic anhydrase is used to convert carbonic acid (bicarbonate + H⁺ion) to carbon dioxide and water in the proximal convoluted tubule of the kidney. It also performs the reverse reaction converting water and carbon dioxide into carbonic acid. Carbonic anhydrase is required for the reabsorption of bicarbonate. Acetazolamide use results in reduced absorption of bicarbonate from the proximal convoluted tubule.

Acetazolamide is used to treat glaucoma and as prophylaxis to prevent mountain sickness. Due to it creating an osmotic diuresis it causes hyponatraemia and hypokalaemia. It also causes a metabolic acidosis (with a normal anion gap) and alkalinisation of the urine, which can cause precipitation of calcium salts and formation of renal stones.

Renal tubular acidosis (RTA) type 1 is where there is poor excretion of H^+ ions in the distal convoluted tubule. RTA type 2 is where there is poor reabsorption of bicarbonate in the proximal convoluted tubule, and this can be caused by acetazolamide. RTA type 4 is due to hyporeninaemic hypoaldosteronism and causes both hyperkalaemia and a metabolic acidosis.

16. D
Indinavir sulphate

Indinavir sulphate is a protease inhibitor used to treat HIV. It is relatively insoluble and therefore can crystallise in the urinary tract to form calculi. It is the only type of stone that doesn't show up on a CT scan. The only other reason that a stone wouldn't be seen is if it is very small and therefore missed by the CT slices that are taken during the imaging.

All other stones: calcium oxalate, calcium phosphate, struvite, urate and cystine can be seen on a CT KUB.

Loop diuretics can increase excretion of calcium and thus may lead to calcium stones forming.

Acetazolamide causes alkalinisation of the urine and precipitation of calcium salts.

Alfacalcidol could lead to hypercalcaemia and therefore increased renal excretion of calcium and renal calculi.

Overuse of laxatives such as senna and persistent diarrhoea has been linked to renal calculi formation. This is because diarrhoea leads to excess ammonium ion secretion and this increases the pH of urine. As a result uric acid binds to ammonium to form ammonium acid urate crystals.

17. B
Diclofenac suppository

This patient is suffering from renal colic. This classically presents with loin pain, nausea and vomiting, dysuria and haematuria. Non-steroidal anti-inflammatory drugs (NSAIDs) are seen as the best form of pain relief. This patient would be unable to take oral medication, and also NSAIDs given as either a suppository or intramuscular injection would relieve the pain faster. Therefore diclofenac suppository is the correct answer.

Naproxen is also an NSAID but the oral route of administration is less suitable in this patient, because he is vomiting.

Intravenous paracetamol may be considered if NSAIDs were contraindicated but wouldn't be first line.

Opiates such as morphine or co-codamol (codeine and paracetamol) can worsen the nausea and vomiting and therefore are not given.

18. D
Schistosomiasis

Schistosomia haematobium is a trematode, which enters the bladder and causes frequency, haematuria, haematospermia and incontinence. If untreated there is scarring of the bladder and an increased risk of squamous cell carcinoma. It is the most common cause of squamous cell carcinoma of the bladder.

The other options are all risk factors for transitional cell carcinoma of the bladder. Working in the rubber industry with aromatic amines, or working as a hairdresser with alanine dyes are both

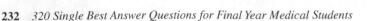

occupational risk factors. Smoking is also a risk factor that hasn't been listed above. Cyclophosphamide is an alkylating agent used in chemotherapy regimes and in immunosuppression. One of its side effects is haemorrhagic cystitis. It can also increase the risk of bladder cancer. It should be given with MESNA to prevent the development of haemorrhagic cystitis.

19. A
Tolterodine

This patient has developed urge incontinence, also known as overactive bladder syndrome. This is caused by the sudden uncontrolled contraction of the detrusor muscle, which causes complete emptying of the bladder. First line treatment is to use a muscarinic antagonist such as tolterodine or oxybutinin. This acts to block the muscarnic receptors on the detrusor muscle and reduce uncontrolled contractions. It helps to treat both urinary urgency and frequency.

Topical oestriol cream is prescribed to patients who have gone through the menopause and have developed vaginitis, as a result of low oestrogen levels. This can cause urge incontinence and also an increased risk of urinary tract infections. However this patient is young, and hasn't had any vaginal bleeding or dyspareunia. Therefore it is unlikely she has developed vaginitis.

Duloxetine is a serotonin-norepinephrine reuptake inhibitor (SNRI), which can be prescribed to treat stress incontinence, and a Burch coloposuspension is a surgical procedure used to treat stress incontinence. Stress incontinence would often have a history of multiple childbirths. It is caused by the leakage of urine from an incompetent sphincter whenever there is an increase in intra-abdominal pressure, such as if a patient coughs, laughs or strains. Only small volumes of urine leak out, as opposed to large volumes in urge incontinence. First line treatment is pelvic floor exercises.

Doxazosin is an alpha-adrenoceptor antagonist used to treat benign prostatic hyperplasia and is a third line treatment for hypertension. It acts by relaxing and dilating the urethra and ureters to allow urine to pass through. One of its listed side effects is incontinence.

9"x6"
b3668_02-Endocrine.indd 45
b3668 320 Single Best Answer Questions for Final Year Medical Students
23-Aug-19 6:

Renal and Urology Answers **233**

20. D
Teratoma

This patient has a testicular tumour, which would typically present with a painless, hard testicular lump. Teratomas are most common in patients who are between 20–30 years old. Their associated tumour makers are alpha-fetoprotein and beta-human chorionic gonadotrophin. They respond well to chemotherapy.

Seminomas are most common between 30–65 years old. They are associated with a raised lactate dehydrogenase and respond well to radiotherapy.

Haematocoeles are a collection of blood in the tunica vaginalis and often follow a history of trauma. They cause a fluctuant lump, which doesn't transluminate.

Hydrocoeles are a collection of fluid in the tunica vaginalis. They can be primary and associated with a patent processus vaginalis, or secondary to a tumour, trauma or infection. They form a fluctuant mass, which does transluminate.

A varicocele is dilated veins in the pampiniform plexus, which has the appearance of 'a bag of worms'.

21. A
Haemoglobin

Normally in chronic kidney disease patients become anaemic due to reduced production of erythropoietin. However in polycystic kidney disease there is production of erythropoietin from the multiple cysts that form in the kidneys. Therefore these patients are less likely to become anaemic.

All other options are affected. A lack of vitamin D production leads to secondary and eventually tertiary hyperparathyroidism. Therefore there is a raised parathyroid hormone level. Serum phosphate and urate are both increased due to a lack of excretion from the kidneys.

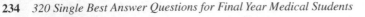

22. C
Candesartan

This patent has developed proteinuria as a result of nephrotic syndrome. Proteinuria is best treated with an angiotensin converting enzyme (ACE) inhibitor or an angiotensin II receptor blocker such as candesartan. Patients with diabetes mellitus who develop proteinuria should also be treated with these drugs. They are shown to reduce proteinuria and improve patients' long-term prognosis.

Human albumin solution can be used to replace albumin, but is most commonly used in patients with liver cirrhosis, who develop ascites. Patients with liver cirrhosis develop hypoalbuminaemia because their liver is no longer producing albumin, therefore human albumin solution can be used to replace it. Human albumin solution would not reduce loss of albumin via the kidneys.

Amiloride is a potassium sparing diuretic. It acts by inhibiting the epithelial sodium channel (ENaC). Its mechanism is different to spironolactone, which is an aldosterone receptor antagonist. Therefore amiloride doesn't cause gynaecomastia.

Bumetanide is a loop diuretic and indapamide is a thiazide-like diuretic used to treat hypertension. Neither of these are effective at reducing proteinuria.

23. B
Transrectal ultrasound and biopsy of the prostate

This patient has an underlying diagnosis of prostate cancer. This presents with storage symptoms (urinary frequency, urgency, nocturia and incontinence) and voiding symptoms (hesitancy, poor stream, post micturition dribbling and pis-en-deux). This patient may also have bone metastases because of his recent weight loss and back pain. However a diagnosis of prostate cancer must be confirmed first and it can only be confirmed by use of a transrectal ultrasound and biopsy of the prostate.

Magnetic resonance imaging (MRI) scan of the prostate may be used as part of staging the cancer, along with a computed tomography (CT) scan of the chest and abdomen. However this would only occur once a formal diagnosis has been made.

Prostate specific antigen (PSA) is a non-specific tumour marker. It can be raised in many scenarios such as benign prostatic hyperplasia, prostatitis, urinary tract infections, post rectal examination, and post intense exercise. Therefore it cannot be used in isolation to make a diagnosis. It's best use is to monitor treatment and also to screen for recurrence.

Serum calcium, phosphate and alkaline phosphatase (ALP) levels would be useful in this patient as we suspect there may be metastases in the spine. However, this wouldn't confirm the underlying diagnosis.

Cystoscopy would be useful if we suspected bladder cancer, but has no role in the diagnosis of prostate cancer.

24. D
Penicillamine

This patient has developed membranous nephropathy. This is the most common cause of nephrotic syndrome in adults. It is diagnosed by use of a renal biopsy which shows thickening of the basement membrane and deposition of both IgG and C3 in the basement membrane. It can be idiopathic or caused by infections (hepatitis B, syphilis, and leprosy), drugs (penicillamine, gold and captopril) or autoimmune diseases (rheumatoid arthritis, systemic lupus erythematosus [SLE] and autoimmune thyroid disease).

Methotrexate doesn't affect the kidneys. Its main side effects are myelosuppression, megaloblastic anaemia, pulmonary fibrosis, hepatic fibrosis and oral ulcers.

Sulfasalazine is a 5-aminosalicylic acid (5-ASA) drug used to treat rheumatoid arthritis and inflammatory bowel disease. It can affect the kidneys by causing an interstitial nephritis. Other side effects include reversible oligospermia, hepatitis, pancreatitis and blood dyscrasias.

Naproxen is a non-steroidal anti-inflammatory drug (NSAID) that can affect the kidneys by causing pre-renal acute kidney injury, interstitial nephritis and minimal change glomerulonephritis. Other side effects include peptic ulceration.

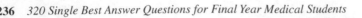

> Leflunomide is an immunomodulatory drug that inhibits dihydroorotate dehydrogenase (which is involved in pyrimidine synthesis). Its side effects include diarrhoea, raised blood pressure and respiratory tract infections. It is also teratogenic in females and males who are trying to conceive.

25. B
1 litre of 0.9% saline STAT

This patient has developed rhabdomyolysis as a result of his prolonged seizure. The skeletal muscle breakdown leads to myoglobin being released into the blood stream. Myoglobin is nephrotoxic. It precipitates in the glomeruli and renal tubules causing obstruction. First line treatment is intravenous fluid rehydration to prevent acute kidney injury. Haemodialysis may be required, but fluid rehydration would occur first. Intravenous sodium bicarbonate can be given to alkalinise the urine and thus stabilise the myoglobin in a less toxic form.

Other complications of rhabdomyolysis include hyperkalaemia (which may require treatment with intravenous insulin and 50% dextrose). However the potassium result has not been given in the stem above, so until it is obtained the priority is rehydration. Other metabolic imbalances include hyperphosphataemia, hypocalcaemia and raised serum urate.

Important causes of rhabdomyolysis include ischaemia (myocardial infarction, embolism), trauma (crush injuries, prolonged immobilisation after falling, burns), and drugs (statins, fibrates, heroin, ecstasy and neuroleptic malignant syndrome caused by antipsychotic drugs).

26. A
Aspirin

Salicylate poisoning can be treated with dialysis. The first line treatment is to give intravenous sodium bicarbonate. This is used to correct any metabolic acidosis, and also alkalinisation of the urine aids

9"x6"
b3668_02-Endocrine.indd 49
b3668   320 Single Best Answer Questions for Final Year Medical Students
23-Aug-19 6

the excretion of salicylates. If this treatment is ineffective, the salicylate levels are extremely high, there is severe acidosis, patients develop seizures or are in heart or renal failure then haemodialysis is used. Drugs that can be removed by haemodialysis include barbiturates, lithium, alcohol, salicylates and theophylline. They are commonly remembered using the 'BLAST' acronym.

Paracetamol overdose is treated with N-acetylcystine.

Amitriptyline binds strongly to plasma proteins and therefore cannot be removed by haemodialysis. An overdose is treated with intravenous sodium bicarbonate.

Diazepam is a benzodiazepine. Often an overdose in one of these drugs is treated conservatively by monitoring the patient. If the patient goes into respiratory depression then flumazenil can be used as an antidote. However flumazenil can provoke seizures, so the preferred management is to monitor the patient until they fully recover.

Propranolol is a beta-blocker. Any overdose of a beta-blocker can cause complete heart block and severe bradycardia. The antidote often used is glucagon. Other drugs commonly given in a decompensated bradycardia include atropine, adrenaline and isoprenaline. Patients with an irreversible bradycardia often require transcutaneous pacing until a permanent pacemaker can be fitted.

27. D
Tacrolimus

Tacrolimus is a calcineurin inhibitor, and belongs to the same group of drugs as ciclosporin. It is known to cause drug induced type 2 diabetes mellitus. This woman has a raised fasting glucose and HbA1c, which is most likely to be due to tacrolimus therapy. Its other side effects include gum hypertrophy, tremor, increased blood pressure, nephrotoxicity, increased risk of skin cancer and lymphoma. Prednisolone is the other immunosuppressive drug that can cause insulin resistance, but it is not listed as an option.

Other drugs commonly used following a kidney transplant are mycophenolate motefil and basiliximab. Mycophenolate motefil is an anti-proliferative agent and its side effects include severe diarrhoea and gastrointestinal bleeding. Basiliximab is a monoclonal antibody that binds to a subunit of the IL-2 receptor on activated T-cells and prevents receptor signalling. Like all immunosuppressive drugs it causes an increased risk of infection.

Mercaptopurine is the active form of azathioprine. Azathioprine is a pro-drug and is metabolised to form mercaptopurine. Its side effects include abdominal pain, darkening of the skin, pancreatitis and myelosuppression.

Cyclophosphamide is an alkylating agent. Its main side effect is haemorrhagic cystitis, but this can be prevented by the use of MESNA.

28. C
Eosinophilic granulomatosis with polyangiitis

Eosinophilic granulomatosis with polyangiitis, also known as Churg-Strauss syndrome, is a small vessel P-ANCA positive myeloperoxidase (MPO) positive, vasculitis. It can cause pulmonary-renal syndrome, which presents with haemoptysis and haematuria. This patient has developed nephritic syndrome and acute kidney injury as a result of a rapidly progressive glomerulonephritis. A renal biopsy would show a crescentic glomerulonephritis. Other features of eosinophilic granulomatosis with polyangiitis include asthma, nasal polyps, eosinophilia and mononeuritis multiplex.

Microscopic polyangiitis is also a small vessel P-ANCA positive vasculitis. It also presents with pulmonary-renal syndrome, but doesn't cause an eosinophilia.

Granulomatosis with polyangiitis, also known as Wegener's granulomatosis, is a small vessel C-ANCA positive, proteinase 3 (PR3) positive, vasculitis. It presents with pulmonary-renal syndrome, sinusitis, epistaxis, saddle shaped nose, scleritis, uveitis, vasculitic rash and arthritis.

Anti-glomerular basement membrane disease, also known as Goodpasture's syndrome, is a small vessel ANCA negative vasculitis caused by antibodies against collagen type IV, which can be found in the basement membrane of the glomerulus and in the lungs. It therefore also presents with a pulmonary-renal syndrome. The antibodies are also known as anti-glomerular basement membrane (GBM) antibodies.

Kawasaki disease is a small to medium vessel vasculitis, which most commonly occurs in children. It presents with a fever, bilateral non-purulent conjunctivitis, cervical lymphadenopathy (>1.5 cm diameter), strawberry tongue, dry fissured lips, vasculitic rash, palmar erythema, desquamation of fingers and toes, and arthralgia.

29. C
Bilateral renal artery stenosis

Angiotensin converting enzyme (ACE) inhibitors cause vasodilation of the efferent glomerular arteriole and therefore ACE inhibitors lead to a reduced glomerular filtration rate, by decreasing the arteriole pressure within the glomerulus. In renal artery stenosis, vasoconstriction of the efferent arteriole is crucial in maintaining the glomerular filtration. Therefore in bilateral renal artery stenosis use of an ACE inhibitor can cause acute kidney injury and lead to flash pulmonary oedema, which is what this patent has presented with. Flash pulmonary oedema presents with rapid onset and causes cough, dyspnea, orthopnea and bilateral fine inspiratory crackles. An arterial blood gas would show type 1 respiratory failure.

Other causes of flash pulmonary oedema include acute myocardial infarction, acute mitral regurgitation heroin and cocaine use.

Acquired angioedema is caused by an acquired deficiency in C1 esterase. It presents similarly to hereditary angioedema, but occurs later on in life. An attack can be precipitated by use of ACE inhibitors as these also inhibit breakdown of bradykinin. The build up of bradykinin activates the compliment system. Normally this over activation would be controlled by the C1-inhibitor (C1 esterase), however in angioedema it is not, resulting in tissue swelling, stridor, urticaria and abdominal pain.

Asthma would present with dyspnea, wheeze, chest tightness, cough and it can be precipitated by beta-blockers and non-steroidal anti-inflammatory drugs (NSAIDs), but not by ACE inhibitors.

Acute urinary obstruction would present with suprapubic pain, and an inability to pass urine. The bladder would be palpable and dull to percussion. It could cause hydronephrosis and acute kidney injury. It can be precipitated by drugs such as anticholinergics, tricyclic antidepressants and alcohol. Other precipitants include post-operative pain, constipation, infection, spinal cord compression, cauda equina syndrome, benign prostatic hyperplasia and prostate cancer.

Congestive cardiac failure would present with pulmonary oedema due to left sided heart failure and also ankle swelling, hepatomegaly and a raised jugular venous pressure (JVP) due to right sided heart failure. Also ACE inhibitors wouldn't precipitate heart failure; instead the symptoms would improve. Precipitants for decompensated heart failure include non-compliance with medication, increased fluid intake, acute myocardial infarction, arrhythmias, valvular disease, myocarditis, sepsis, tension penumothorax, cardiac tamponade, drugs (non-dihydropyridine calcium channel blockers, NSAIDs, pioglitazone, clozapine, trastuzumab and anthracyclines).

30. C
Hydronephrosis

This patient has developed urinary obstruction and as a result developed hydronephrosis. The patient's bladder is palpable. This patient is not complaining of any pain so it is likely that this is chronic urinary obstruction. The build-up of urine has caused hydronephosis, which presents with enlarged kidneys and renal failure.

Any cause of obstruction can lead to hydronephrosis. Causes include renal calculi, benign prostatic hyperplasia, malignancy (bladder cancer, prostate cancer and urethral cancer), urethral stenosis and retroperitoneal fibrosis.

Other causes of bilaterally enlarged kidneys include polycystic kidney disease, bilateral renal cell carcinomas, amyloidosis and tuberous sclerosis (due to renal angiomyolipomata and cysts).

Polycystic kidney disease would present with renal failure much earlier in life. Other features would include liver cysts, berry aneurysms (leading to subarachnoid haemorrhage) and mitral valve prolapse.

Amyloidosis would cause other systemic signs and symptoms such as hepatomegaly, splenomegaly, restrictive cardiomyopathy, mononeuritis multiplex, autonomic neuropathy, macroglossia, nephrotic syndrome and periorbital purpura.

Bilateral renal artery stenosis would result in both kidneys becoming atrophic and smaller than normal.

Lung cancer classically metastasises to the bone, brain, liver and adrenal glands. It wouldn't cause an enlarged bladder. It would also present with cough, dyspnea, chest pain and weight loss.

9"x6" b3668   320 Single Best Answer Questions for Final Year Medical Students
b3668_02-Endocrine.indd 55
23-Aug-19 6:

Respiratory Questions

1. An 18-year-old male is due to be admitted to the respiratory ward following a severe asthma attack. During his transition to the ward from the emergency department he develops sudden worsening shortness of breath, and pleuritic chest pain. Which of the following investigations would confirm the underlying cause of his new onset dyspnea?

A. Computed tomography pulmonary angiogram (CTPA)
B. Peak flow measurements
C. Chest X-ray
D. Arterial blood gas
E. Echocardiogram

2. A 70-year-old frail woman who is currently recovering from a bout of left leg cellulitis was brought into hospital following sudden onset sharp chest pain, dyspnea, cough and haemoptysis. Her routine bloods are below:

Haemoglobin: 81 g/L
White cell count: 10.1×10^9/L
Serum sodium: 141 mmol/L
Serum potassium: 5.5 mmol/L
Serum urea: 21 mg/dL
Serum creatinine: 190 µmol/L

Which of the following investigations should be used to confirm the underlying diagnosis?

A. Computed tomography pulmonary angiogram (CTPA)
B. Ventilation/perfusion scan
C. D-dimer
D. Chest X-ray
E. Echocardiogram

3. A 23-year-old lady is being treated for a severe asthma attack. So far she has received back-to-back salbutamol and ipratropium nebulisers and oral prednisolone. On examination her chest is now clear and she has a fine tremor. Her arterial blood gas (ABG) samples show normal gases but a rising lactate. Which of the following is likely to be causing the rising lactate levels?

A. Underlying bacterial pneumonia
B. Myocardial infarction
C. Exhaustion
D. Salbutamol toxicity
E. Pneumothorax

4. An elderly man presented to clinic with worsening breathlessness and a persistent cough. On his chest X-ray there is bilateral hilar lymphadenopathy, eggshell calcification of the hila and a diffuse nodular pattern in the upper lobes. What is the most likely underlying diagnosis?

A. Sarcoidosis
B. Lymphoma
C. Silicosis
D. Asbestosis
E. Idiopathic pulmonary fibrosis

5. A 54-year-old man presents to hospital following a one-week history of massive haemoptysis. His chest X-ray shows a target shaped lesion in the left upper lobe. It is a caseating lesion with a white centre. His Mantoux test is positive, but his interferon gamma release assay (IGRA) test is negative. What is the most likely diagnosis?

A. Mycobacterium tuberculosis
B. Aspergilloma
C. Granulomatosis with polyangiitis
D. Sarcoidosis
E. Bronchiectasis

6. A 32-year-old male presents to his doctor with chest pain. The pain is worse on inspiration and is described as sharp. On examination there is swelling and localised tenderness of the costal cartilages; just left of the sternum. What is the most likely underlying diagnosis?

A. Tiezte syndrome
B. Bolhorm disease
C. Costochondritis
D. Bone metastases
E. Pneumothorax

7. An 85-year-old non-smoker who spent most of his life working on the shipping yards presents to his doctor with a dull chest pain, weight loss and worsening breathlessness. On examination he has finger clubbing and reduced chest expansion on the left side. The left base is dull to percussion, has reduced breath sounds and reduced vocal resonance. Which of the following best describes the pathological process behind this patient's symptoms?

A. Caseating granuloma formation
B. Metastatic tumour originating from the pleural epithelial cells
C. Extensive scarring and thickening of the pleura
D. Metastatic adenocarcinoma originating from the lung tissue
E. Deposition of rheumatoid factor in the intersitium

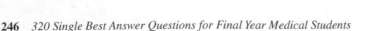

8. An elderly gentleman who has smoked cigarettes most of his life presents to his doctor with worsening ankle swelling. On examination his doctor notices that he has a left parasternal heave, bilateral pitting oedema up to his knees and a raised jugular venous pressure. His recent lung function tests showed an obstructive picture and his arterial blood gas on room air showed a PaO_2 of 7.6 kPa. Which of the following would improve this patient's life expectancy the most?

A. Prophylactic antibiotics
B. Carbocisteine
C. Furosemide
D. Long term low dose oral prednisolone
E. Long term oxygen therapy

9. A young lady presents to her doctor with a dry cough and pain in both her knees and ankles. On examination she has painful purple nodules on both of her shins and swollen knee and ankle joints bilaterally. A chest X-ray shows bilateral hilar lymphadenopathy. Which of the following is the most appropriate treatment regime for this patient?

A. Oral naproxen
B. Oral prednisolone
C. Intravenous methylprednisolone
D. Intravenous infliximab
E. Oral rifampicin, isoniazid, pyrazinamide and ethambutol

10. A patient being treated for asthma develops white furry patches on her tongue and the sides of her mouth. Which of the following is the most appropriate treatment regime for this patient?

A. Stop the beclometasone for four days
B. Switch beclometasone to salmetrol permanently
C. Reduce the beclometasone dose and prescribe oral fluconazole
D. Maintain same beclometasone dose and prescribe oral aciclovir
E. Maintain same beclometasone dose and prescribe nystatin suspension

11. A patient with a history of chronic obstructive pulmonary disease (COPD) has a DLCO (diffusing capacity factor of the lung for carbon monoxide) as part of a set of investigations to evaluate his lung function. Which of the following would be responsible for a raised DLCO in this patient?

A. Pulmonary hypertension
B. Right sided heart failure
C. Polycythaemia
D. Bullae formation
E. Pulmonary embolism

12. A young patient with a background of asthma presents to hospital short of breath. Following treatment with back to back salbutamol and ipratropium nebulizers, intravenous hydrocortisone and intravenous magnesium, the patient is still extremely short of breath. His latest arterial blood gas (ABG) taken on 15 litres of supplementary oxygen shows the following:

pH: 7.29
$PaCO_2$:   7.01 kPa
PaO_2:   6.2 kPa

Which of the following is the most appropriate next step in this patient's management?

A. Continuous positive airway pressure (CPAP) ventilation
B. Bilevel positive airway pressure (BiPAP) ventilation
C. Endotracheal intubation and mechanical ventilation
D. Intravenous salbutamol
E. Intravenous aminophylline

13. A 24-year-old patient recovering from pneumonia relapses with a recurrent fever. She reports severe left sided pleurtic chest pain and on examination she has a temperature of 39 degrees Celcius, finger clubbing and reduced air entry and vocal resonance at the base of her left lung. Which of the following is the most likely cause of this patients relapse?

A. Septicaemia
B. Empyema
C. Antibiotic resistance
D. Underlying bronchial carcinoma
E. Tuberculosis infection

14. A 34-year-old patient presents to hospital with breathlessness and sudden onset sharp chest pain. A chest X-ray shows a pneumothorax with a rim of 1 cm. He has no significant past medical history. Which of the following is the most appropriate management of this patient's presentation?

A. Discharge home
B. Monitor for 24 hours and repeat a chest X-ray before discharge
C. Aspiration of the pneumothorax
D. Insertion of a chest drain
E. Insert a cannula through the intercostal muscles

15. A farmer is brought into hospital a few hours after finishing work with a fever, rigors, headache and dyspnea. His chest X-ray shows bilateral hilar lymphadenopathy and upper zone consolidation. Which of the following investigations would be most useful in this patient?

A. Specific IgE to pollen
B. Serum precipitants to thermophilic fungi
C. Aspergillus skin test
D. Blood cultures
E. Lung biopsy

16. A patient with severe chronic obstructive pulmonary disease (COPD) was recently started on theophylline. He is already on maximal doses of salmetrol, salbutamol, tiotropium and beclometasone. Which of the following electrolyte imbalances is his doctor most concerned about?

A. Hyperkalaemia
B. Hypokalaemia
C. Hypercalcaemia
D. Hypocalcaemia
E. Hypophosphataemia

17. A 20-year-old man who has been smoking 20 cigarettes a day for the last 2 years presents to his doctor with worsening shortness of breath. His lung function tests show a forced expiratory volume in one second (FEV$_1$) of 65% predicted, a forced vital capacity (FVC) of 90% predicted and an FEV$_1$/FVC ratio of 72%. A high resolution computed tomography (HRCT) scan of the chest shows lower lobe panacinar emphysema. Which of the following is the most likely diagnosis?

A. Asthma
B. Cystic fibrosis
C. Chronic obstructive pulmonary disease (COPD)
D. Alpha-1-antitrypsin deficiency
E. Pulmonary fibrosis

18. A 60-year-old man with a history of recurrent epistaxis presents to hospital with a fever, polyarthralgia, dyspnea, cough and haemoptysis. On examination he is found to have a non-blanching purpuric rash on his shins. His urine dipstick shows the following:

Blood: +++
Protein: +++

Which of the following antibodies is most likely to be present?

A. Perinuclear anti-neutrophil cytoplasmic antibodies (P-ANCA)
B. Cytoplasmic anti-neutrophil cytoplasmic antibodies (C-ANCA)
C. Anti–glomerular basement membrane (anti-GBM) antibody
D. Anti-double-stranded DNA (anti-dsDNA) antibody
E. Anti-RNP antibodies

19. An 89-year-old woman died alone in her flat. A post-mortem was carried out. Her lungs were found to be heavier than normal and grey in colour. Histology showed raised levels of alveolar neutrophils. Which of the following is the most likely underlying cause of death?

A. Acute respiratory distress syndrome (ARDS)
B. Pneumonia
C. Tuberculosis
D. Chronic obstructive pulmonary disease (COPD) exacerbation
E. Lung cancer

20. A 21-year-old male died recently following a bout of multiple respiratory infections. Prior to this a respiratory consultant was monitoring him due to his lung function tests showing a reduced forced expiratory volume in one second/forced vital capacity (FEV_1/FVC) ratio. He also had type 1 diabetes mellitus. Considering the underlying diagnosis which of the following is most likely to be found in a biopsy of this patient's lungs?

A. Charcot-Laden crystals
B. Panacinar emphysema
C. Centriacinar emphysema
D. Dilated bronchioles
E. Non-caseating granulomas

21. An 85-year-old patient with mild dementia and chronic obstructive pulmonary disease (COPD), which is controlled with seretide and tiotropium inhalers, presents with gradually worsening shortness of breath. Her observations show she is tachypnoeic, tachycardic, normotensive and apyrexial. Her arterial blood gas (ABG) shows the following:

pH: 7.31
$PaCO_2$:   9.1 kPa
PaO_2:   8.0 kPa
Bicarbonate: 30 mmol/L

Her blood tests show a normal white cell count (WCC) and normal C-reactive protein (CRP).

Two weeks ago she was discharged from hospital, and her ABG then showed:

pH: 7.36
$PaCO_2$:   6.5 kPa
PaO_2:   9.0 kPa
Bicarbonate: 31 mmol/L

Which of the following is the most likely cause of her symptoms?

A. Infective exacerbation of COPD
B. Non-compliance with medication
C. Pulmonary embolism
D. Pneumothorax
E. Pulmonary oedema

22. A pregnant lady presents to hospital with sudden onset sharp pleuritic chest pain. She has had one episode of haemoptysis. Her observations are normal. On examination of her chest vesicular breath sounds can be heard. Her left calf is swollen and tender. A venous doppler scan is unable to compress the underlying veins, and confirms there is a reduced venous blood flow. Which of the following should occur next?

A. Computed tomography pulmonary angiogram (CTPA)
B. Ventilation/perfusion scan
C. Start treatment dose of dalteparin
D. Start treatment dose of dalteparin and initiate warfarin therapy
E. Start warfarin therapy

23. A 40-year-old man is found barely conscious by his neighbour, following an attempted suicide. He was found in his garage after inhaling fumes from the exhaust pipe of his car. On examination he is cyanosed, tachycardic, tachypnoeic and has bilateral fine inspiratory crepitations throughout his chest. Which of the following forms of ventilation is most useful in this patient?

A. 24% oxygen via a venturi mask
B. Nebulised salbutamol and 15 L/min of oxygen via a non-rebreath mask
C. Bilevel positive airway pressure (BiPAP) and high flow oxygen
D. Continuous positive airway pressure (CPAP) and high flow oxygen
E. Nasal intermittent positive pressure ventilation (NIPPV)

24. An elderly lady is brought into hospital. Her daughter states that the patient is confused, and drowsier than normal. She states that her mother hasn't left her cottage for a few days and has spent a lot of time sitting in front of an open fire. Apart from mild tachypnoea her observations are normal and on examination the only findings were that her hands were warm and pink in colour and both pupils were dilated. Which of the following treatments should be given?

A. Ceftriaxone
B. Amoxicillin and clarithromycin
C. Naloxone
D. Sodium bicarbonate
E. 15 litres of oxygen via a non-rebreath mask

25. A 75-year-old male developed a cough, haemoptysis, and dyspnea and over the past two months experienced unintentional weight loss. He also describes having shooting pains down his left arm. On examination he has finger clubbing. His left arm has weakness throughout and loss of sensation in all dermatomes. His right arm is completely normal. Which of the following findings would be most consistant with the underlying diagnosis?

A. Erythema nodosum
B. New pan-systolic murmur
C. Haematuria
D. Unilaterally constricted pupil
E. Stridor

26. A 24-year-old male presents with a fever, dry cough and polyar-thralgia. This was preceded by a period of malaise. On examination of his chest scattered coarse crepitations can be heard. On full exposure his body is covered with symmetrical target lesions. Which of the following findings would be most consistent with the underlying diagnosis?

A. Lobar consolidation seen on a chest X-ray
B. Tramline appearance of the bronchioles seen on a chest X-ray
C. Gram-positive cocci grown in sputum cultures
D. Positive cold direct Coombs test
E. Alpha haemolytic gram-positive diplococcus chains found in blood cultures

27. A 65-year-old lady is brought into hospital due to shortness of breath. She has a worsening cough over the past few days and brought up rust coloured sputum. On examination coarse inspiratory crepitations can be heard at the right base. Which of the following is the most likely cause of this patient's symptoms?

A. Influenza virus
B. Streptococcus pneumoniae
C. Haemophilus influenza
D. Staphylococcus aureus
E. Chlamydophilia psittaci

28. A 45-year-old overweight male attends his general practitioner (GP) appointment with his wife. He is complaining of tiredness, lethargy and irritability. His wife also mentions that he has been falling asleep during the day. His past medical history includes hypertension. Which of the following should occur next in this patient's management?

A. Short course of zopiclone to be taken at night
B. Trial of antidepressants
C. Computed tomography (CT) scan of the head, neck and chest
D. Sleep studies
E. Early morning arterial blood gas samples

29. Which of the following best describes the pathological process behind the formation of a para-pneumonic pleural effusion?

A. Decreased oncotic pressure
B. Impaired lymphatic drainage
C. Increased capillary permeability
D. Destruction of the visceral pleura
E. Elevated hydrostatic pressure

30. A 75-year-old man with known chronic obstructive pulmonary disease (COPD) is prescribed antibiotics by his doctor to treat a chest infection. He is also taking seretide, tiotropium, theophylline, and prednisolone regularly and salbutamol when required. A few days later he develops abdominal pain, nausea, vomiting and diarrhoea. On examination he is tachycardic and his initial blood tests show a high theophylline level. Which of the following antibiotics was he prescribed by his doctor?

A. Amoxicillin
B. Sulfamethoxazole/trimethoprim
C. Erythromycin
D. Rifampicin
E. Doxycycline

Respiratory Answers

1. C
Chest X-ray

This patient has developed a pneumothorax. Asthmatic patients are at a high risk of developing a pneumothorax and therefore it should always be considered as a cause of worsening breathlessness in these patients. Other patients at a higher risk include those with other lung pathologies (chronic obstructive pulmonary disease (COPD), bronchiectasis, pulmonary fibrosis, lung cancer), and connective tissue diseases (Marfan syndrome and Ehlers-Danlos syndrome). It would present with sudden onset pleuritic chest pain and dyspnea. A chest X-ray can confirm the diagnosis. If it is small and the radiologist is unsure of whether a pneumothorax is present or not, an expiratory film can be requested. This would emphasize the pneumothorax.

CTPA would be used to diagnose a pulmonary embolism. This would present with sudden onset pleuritic chest pain, dyspnea and haemoptysis, but is unlikely in a young patient with no risk factors for venous thromboembolism.

Arterial blood gas and peak flow measurements would be useful in this patient to monitor the severity of the asthma attack, but would not confirm the underlying diagnosis of a pneumothorax. An echocardiogram is of no use in this patient.

2. B
Ventilation/perfusion

This woman has a pulmonary embolism (PE). She has presented with the classic symptoms of a PE, which include sudden onset pleuritic chest pain, dyspnea, and haemoptysis.

Normally a CTPA would be used to confirm the diagnosis as it is the most accurate, however from the blood results it is evident that she is in renal failure and therefore the CTPA would be contraindicated. The contrast used is nephrotoxic and could cause further renal damage.

Her serum urea and creatinine are high, and she is anaemic which could be due to chronic kidney disease. A ventilation/perfusion scan is the next best option and looks for ventilation-perfusion mismatch in the lungs.

A D-dimer can be used to exclude a deep vein thrombosis (DVT) or PE if the likelihood of a DVT or PE is very low. If the D-dimer is negative it excludes a DVT or PE. However the likelihood in this patient is high due to her symptoms and therefore it should not be used. Also the D-dimer is an acute phase protein and therefore is raised in any cause of inflammation such as infection.

An echocardiogram can be used to diagnose a massive PE. In an emergency if the patient has gone into shock and a PE is suspected an echocardiogram can be used. If right sided strain can be seen then the patient is likely to have a PE; if not then a PE can be ruled out. This is used if a patient is too unstable to be put through a computed tomography (CT) scanner.

3. D
Salbutamol toxicity

Nebulised salbutamol can lead to lactic acidosis. The reasons behind this are still unclear, but the most widely accepted theory is that beta-agonists enhance cyclic adenosine monophosphate (cAMP) mediated gluconeogenesis. The increased plasma glucose is converted to pyruvate via glycolysis, which is then converted to lactate. Therefore in patients receiving salbutamol, lactate levels should be monitored. Other side effects include tremor, hypokalaemia, tachycardia and arrhythmias.

An underlying bacterial pneumonia would have caused inspiratory course crepitations on auscultation of the chest. Sepsis is an important cause of lactic acidosis but is unlikely here.

This patient is too young to be having a myocardial infarction. Also there is no report of central crushing chest pain, vomiting or sweating.

Exhaustion can occur in an asthma attack. It is a sign of a life threatening asthma attack. This would lead to a type 2 respiratory failure. In this patient the blood gases have normalised and therefore this is unlikely.

A pneumothorax is always something that should be considered in asthmatic patients, as they are at a higher risk of developing one. However this would present with type 1 respiratory failure rather than a lactic acidosis.

4. C
Silicosis

The first three options all cause bilateral hilar lymphadenopathy, however the eggshell calcification of the hila is more classical of silicosis. This is an occupational disease caused by sandblasting, metal mining and pottery. It causes lung fibrosis, mainly in the upper and middle lobes. Silicosis also increases the chance of patients being infected by Mycobacterium tuberculosis.

Lymphoma wouldn't cause pulmonary fibrosis.

Sarcoidosis is an idiopathic autoimmune multi-system condition caused by non-caseating granulomas. It more commonly affects younger patients and often causes other symptoms such as chest pain, weight loss, arthralgia etc. It can progress to also cause upper lobe fibrosis.

Both asbestosis and idiopathic pulmonary fibrosis cause lower lobe fibrosis.

5. B
Aspergilloma

The main differential diagnoses for massive haemoptysis are: bronchial carcinoma, tuberculosis, lung abscesses, aspergilloma, and bronchiectasis (especially if the patient has a history of cystic fibrosis). In this scenario this patient had a negative IGRA test, meaning he doesn't have latent, or active tuberculosis; but a positive matoux test, which suggests he has either had a previous history of tuberculosis or a Bacillus Calmette–Guérin (BCG) vaccination. Patients with a previous history of tuberculosis are at risk of aspergillomas, because the fungi are able to infect the lung cavities created by the previous tuberculosis infection. The target shaped lesion is classic of an aspergilloma. It also has strongly positive serum precipitins, and some patients have a positive aspergillus skin test. In many cases they are asymptomatic, but can also cause a cough, weight loss and lethargy.

Mycobacterium tuberculosis would cause a positive IGRA test.

Wegener's granulomatosis is a cytoplasmic anti-neutrophil cytoplasmic antibodies (C-ANCA) positive vasculitis, which would cause a multitude of symptoms including haemoptysis. It would also affect the kidneys and upper airways. A chest X-ray would be more likely to show diffuse areas of shadowing rather than a confined lesion.

Sarcoidosis is more likely to show bilateral hilar lymphadenopathy and fibrosis of the upper lobes on a chest X-ray. Also it often gives a negative mantoux test, even if there has been previous exposure to tuberculosis.

Bronchiectasis is permanent dilatation of the terminal bronchioles. Chest X-ray characteristics would include a tramline appearance and ring shadows due to thickened bronchiole walls. Causes of bronchiectasis include infections (tuberculosis, measles, pertussis, recurrent pneumonias), bronchiole obstruction (foreign body, tumour), allergic bronchopulmonary aspergillosis (ABPA), congenital conditions (cystic fibrosis, Kartagener's syndrome, Young's syndrome, primary cilary dyskinesia) and most commonly it is idiopathic.

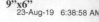

6. A
Tietze syndrome

This is the presence of costochondritis (benign temporary inflammation of the costal cartilage) and swelling of the costal cartilage. If there were no swelling then it would be known as just costochondritis. Bolhorm disease is costochondritis caused by a viral infection, such as Coxsackie B virus. This would be present with coryzal symptoms such as a fever and headache.

Bone metastases are unlikely due to the young age of the patient and also due to the fact there are lots of swellings, which would mean there would have to be lots of metastases to the bone close to the joint. This would be extremely unlikely.

Pneumothorax would present with sudden onset pleuritic chest pain, but wouldn't cause tenderness or swelling of the costal cartilages.

7. B
Metastatic tumour originating from the pleural epithelial cells

This patient has developed a metastatic mesothelioma. This is a malignant proliferation of the pleural cells caused by asbestos exposure. It presents with chest pain, dyspnea, finger clubbing, weight loss, and causes an exudative pleural effusion.

Caseating granuloma formation in the lungs occurs in a tuberculosis infection.

Extensive scarring and thickening of the pleura can occur in asbestosis, but this wouldn't cause a pleural effusion or the extreme weight loss seen here.

A metastatic adenocarcinoma is the most common primary lung tumour in non-smokers. Although this could cause a pleural effusion, a mesothelioma is much more likely in this situation due to the asbestos exposure.

Rheumatoid factor deposition in the interstitium occurs in rheumatoid arthritis and can lead to pulmonary fibrosis. This patient is very old to have developed new onset rheumatoid arthritis and there is no report of joint pains, or other systemic symptoms caused by rheumatoid arthritis.

8. E
Long term oxygen therapy

This gentleman has an underlying diagnosis of chronic obstructive pulmonary disease (COPD), based on his long smoking history and obstructive airways disease. He has also developed cor pulmonale, which is right ventricular failure secondary to pulmonary hypertension resulting from chronic hypoxia. Clinical signs of cor pulmonale include peripheral oedema, a raised JVP and a right ventricular heave.

Long term oxygen therapy has been shown to improve life expectancy in patients with COPD who have a PaO_2 of 7.3–8.0 kPa and pulmonary hypertension.

Carbocisteine is a mucolytic agent, which may help relieve a chronic cough, and help patients clear mucus.

Prophylactic antibiotics may be given to COPD patients who have multiple infective exacerbations, but would not improve the overall prognosis. Furosemide is a loop diuretic that would be used to relieve peripheral oedema in patients that have developed cor pulmonale.

Long term low dose oral prednisolone is likely to result in multiple steroid induced side effects such as osteoporosis, insulin resistance, gastric ulceration and hypertension.

Of the available treatment options, long term oxygen therapy is the only option that has been proven to improve prognosis in patients with COPD and cor pulmonale.

9. A
Oral Naproxen

This lady has Lofgren syndrome, which is a form of acute sarcoidosis. Lofgren syndrome is characterised by a triad of bilateral hilar lymphadenopathy, erythema nodosum and arthritis. It has a good prognosis and often only requires treatment with non-steroidal anti-inflammatory drugs (NSAIDs) such as naproxen.

In patients with sarcoidosis, corticosteroid treatment is only indicated to treat parenchymal lung disease, uveitis, hypercalcaemia, neurosarcoidosis or cardiac sarcoidosis.

Infliximab is a monoclonal antibody that acts against tumor necrosis factor alpha (TNF-α) and is mainly used to treat rheumatoid arthritis and inflammatory bowel disease.

Oral rifampicin, isoniazid, pyrazinamide and ethambutol would be used to treat an active Mycobacterium tuberculosis infection. Although there are many similarities between tuberculosis and sarcoidosis, the above presentation is highly specific for Lofgren syndrome, making it the most likely diagnosis.

10. E
Maintain same beclometasone dose and prescribe nystatin suspension

This patient has developed oral candidiasis as a result of inhaled steroid use. It is important that the patient maintains her current dose of steroids to prevent her from having an asthma attack. Treatment can either be use of a nystatin suspension, amphotericin lozenges or oral fluclonazole for oropharyngeal candidiasis. Prophylaxis would include reviewing inhaler technique, using a spacer to improve inhaler technique and washing her mouth with salt water after using her inhaler.

Salmeterol is a long acting beta-agonist. It is added to patient's therapy if they are already on salbutamol and an inhaled steroid but still have insufficient control. It should never replace the inhaled steroid.

Aciclovir is a guanosine analogue antiviral medication used to treat herpes simplex infections. Aciclovir is incorporated into the viral DNA and prevents viral replication.

11. C
Polycythaemia

DLCO is a measure of the diffusion capacity of the lung, and measures the extent at which carbon monoxide passes from the alveoli into the blood. This is reduced by a decrease in the surface area for gaseous exchange (e.g. bullae formation), hindrance of the alveolar wall (e.g. pulmonary fibrosis), pulmonary hypertension, ventilation/perfusion mismatch (e.g. pulmonary embolism) and anaemia.

It can be increased by asthma, polycythaemia, right to left shunting (e.g. pulmonary haemorrhage and left sided heart failure) and increased pulmonary blood flow (e.g. exercise). Right-sided heart failure alone would not have any effect on the DLCO result.

12. C
Endotracheal intubation and mechanical ventilation

This patient is having a life threatening asthma attack based on the high $PaCO_2$ seen on the most recent arterial blood gas. He has already been treated with medical therapy, but the presence of a normal or high carbon dioxide level on the arterial blood gas is a sign that he is getting tired and will need to be intubated.

Other signs of a life threatening asthma attack are a peak expiratory flow of < 33% of predicted, silent chest, cyanosis, bradycardia, hypotension, exhaustion or confusion.

Continuous positive airway pressure (CPAP) ventilation and bilevel positive airway pressure (BiPAP) ventilation are both contraindicated in asthma. CPAP can be used to treat pulmonary oedema and sleep apnoea, and BiPAP can be used to treat exacerbations of chronic obstructive pulmonary disease (COPD).

Intravenous salbutamol and aminophylline can be used as treatment in patients with asthma exacerbations. However, this patient is showing signs of exhaustion and the most effective way of treating his type 2 respiratory failure is intubation and mechanical ventilation.

13. B
Empyema

Respiratory causes of clubbing are: abscess, bronchiectasis, lung cancer, tuberculosis, empyema and mesothelioma. The complications of pneumonia include abscess formation, empyema, septicaemia, and respiratory failure. An empyema classically presents with a patient who has a resolving pneumonia and develops a recurrent fever and pleuritic chest pain. Aspiration of the pleural fluid would show protein >35 g/L (exudate), pH <7.2, glucose <3.3 mmol/L and raised lactate dehyrdogenase (LDH) (pleural: serum >0.6).

A bronchial carcinoma can increase the risk of developing pneumonia, but this is unlikely due to this patient's young age, and also it wouldn't cause a relapsing fever. All patients should have a repeat chest X-ray once the pneumonia has resolved to look for any underlying cause.

Septicaemia would have presented with this patient being unwell, and would have occurred from the pneumonia. There wouldn't have been any recovery in between, and the patient would have been hypotensive and tachycardic.

Antibiotic resistance may present with a recurring pneumonia, which would typically present with a fever, productive cough and dyspnea. However it wouldn't cause clubbing.

14. C
Aspiration of the pneumothorax

Normally if a patient presents to hospital with their first pneumothorax and the rim is less than 2 cm, they can be discharged. However if they are breathless then they require treatment. The first line treatment is aspiration, and if this doesn't work then a chest drain is inserted.

If a patient has an underlying lung condition causing a secondary pneumothorax, the treatment is slightly different. If the rim is between 1–2 cm then aspiration is used, or if it is greater than 2 cm a chest drain is inserted immediately.

Tension pneumothorax requires a large bore cannula to be inserted into the second intercostal space, mid-clavicular line.

15. B
Serum precipitants to thermophilic fungi

This patient has developed hypersensitivity pneumonitis (also known as extrinsic allergic alveolitis). This is a type III and IV hypersensitivity reaction to organic occupational exposures. It presents with a fever, rigors, myalgia, cough and dyspnea roughly six hours after exposure. The chest X-ray shows bilateral hilar lymphadenopathy and upper zone consolidation acutely; and chronically it causes upper zone fibrosis and honeycombing. Blood tests often show positive serum precipitins and a raised erythrocyte sedimentation rate (ESR). It is treated with oxygen and prednisolone but most importantly by removal of the precipitating factor.

Causes of extrinsic allergic alveolitis include: Micropolyspora faeni and Thermactinomyces vulgaris in farmers, malt worker's lung caused by Aspergillus clavatus, and bird fanciers lung caused by exposure to proteins in bird droppings.

Specific IgE to pollen may help diagnose the cause of asthma and hayfever in some patients.

Aspergillus skin test is used to diagnose allergic bronchopulmonary asperillosis (ABPA), and may also be positive in an aspergilloma.

Blood cultures would help if an infection were suspected.

Lung biopsies are used to confirm a diagnosis of lung cancer.

16. B
Hypokalaemia

This patient is already on two β-agonists. One of the side effects of these is hypokalaemia, because they act to drive potassium ions into cells. Therefore salbutamol can be used to treat hyperkalaemia. Theophylline is also a cause of hypokalaemia, and this effect is increased when used with β-agonists.

17. D
Alpha-1-antitrypsin deficiency

Alpha-1-antitrypsin is a serine protease inhibitor, which protects the lungs against damage from neutrophil elastase. Alpha-1-antitrypsin deficiency is a genetic disorder that results in reduced production of alpha-1-antitrypsin. There is damage to the lungs as a result of over activity of neutrophil elastase. Patients develop emphysema at a young age and can also develop liver cirrhosis. Classically the emphysema is panacinar and in the lower lobes. The condition is diagnosed by testing for serum alpha-1-antitrypsin levels, and treatment is mainly supportive, encouraging smoking cessation and in some patients supplementary alpha-1-antitrypsin pooled from human plasma can be given. The lung function tests would show an obstructive picture. Other causes of obstructive airways disease include asthma, COPD and bronchiectasis.

This patient is too young to have developed COPD and also has a very short smoking history. Most patients with COPD are > 35 years old. The pattern of emphysema in COPD is also different. It is centriacinar and initially affects the upper lobes.

Cystic fibrosis is an autosomal recessive condition caused by mutations in the gene for the cystic fibrosis transmembrane conductance regulator (CFTR) protein. It results in multiple chest infections and bronchiectasis, which would be seen on the HRCT scan of the chest.

Although asthma also causes obstructive airways disease, it would not result in the emphysematous changes that are seen on the HRCT scan.

Pulmonary fibrosis would be unlikely in this patient because of his age and also because his lung function tests have shown an obstructive picture, rather than the restrictive picture that would be seen in pulmonary fibrosis.

18. B
Cytoplasmic anti-neutrophil cytoplasmic antibodies (C-ANCA)

This patient has granulomatosis with polyangiitis, which is also known as Wegener's granulomatosis. It is a small vessel, C-ANCA positive vasculitis and presents with epistaxis, a saddle shaped nose, scleritis, uveitis, a vasculitic rash, and pulmonary-renal syndrome. It causes a rapidly progressive glomerulonephritis and therefore can also cause haematuria and proteinuria.

P-ANCA may be present in eosinophilic granulomatosis with polyangiitis (also known as Churg-Strauss syndrome), microscopic polyangiitis, ulcerative colitis and primary sclerosing cholangitis.

Eosinophilic granulomatosis with polyangiitis and microscopic polyangiitis can both cause pulmonary-renal syndrome, but epistaxis makes granulomatosis with polyangiitis more likely in this case.

Anti-GBM antibody is present in anti-GBM disease, also known as Goodpasture syndrome. These antibodies attack the type IV collage in the basement membrane present in the lungs and kidneys, and also cause pulmonary-renal syndrome.

Anti-dsDNA antibody is present in systemic lupus erythematosus (SLE) and anti-RNP antibodies are present in mixed connective tissue diseases.

19. B
Pneumonia

This patient died of a bacterial pneumonia. This is evident in the increased levels of alveolar neutrophils. Furthermore the lungs are heavier due to the neutrophil infiltration and consolidation. The grey colour is referred to as grey hepatisation. First there is congestion, which is characterised by neutrophil infiltration; then there is red hepatisation, which is due to vascular congestion causing red cell extravasation, and finally there is grey hepatisation where the red cells disintegrate leaving just the neutrophils behind.

In ARDS there would be hyaline membrane thickening seen on histology.

Tuberculosis would lead to multiple caseating granulomas being seen on histology in the apices of the lungs. There is also likely to be cavities and evidence of fibrosis.

COPD is a combination of chronic bronchitis and emphysema, which is seen on histology as multiple bullae formed as a result of alveolar wall destruction.

Lung cancer would be seen as a mass, and histology would show malignant cells that could be characterised as squamous cell carcinoma, adenocarcinoma, small cell or large cell carcinomas.

20. D
Dilated bronchioles

This patient has cystic fibrosis, which is caused by an autosomal recessive mutation in the chloride channel, leading to excess mucus production. This causes lots of infections and results in bronchiectasis (permanently dilated terminal bronchioles). Cystic fibrosis also causes pancreatic insufficiency, which results in type 1 diabetes mellitus, steatorrhea and fat soluble vitamin deficiencies. Vitamin D deficiency leads to osteomalacia. Other complications include liver cirrhosis, gallstones and male infertility.

Charcot-Leyden crystals are created by eosinophils and found in asthma, and parasitic infections.

Panacinar emphysema occurs in alpha-1-antitrypsin deficiency. This condition leads to increased protease activity and destruction of the alveoli and terminal bronchioles. It mainly affects the lower lobes.

Centriacinar emphysema occurs in chronic obstructive pulmonary disease (COPD) and is a result of inflammation caused by cigarette smoke. There is up regulation of the protease enzymes (especially neutrophil elastase).

Non-caseating granulomas occur in sarcoidosis, and these would mainly affect the upper lobes of the lungs.

21. B
Non-compliance with medication

This patient has presented with a non-infective exacerbation of COPD. The reasons for this are she has worsening shortness of breath and type 2 respiratory failure on her ABG. The raised bicarbonate is likely to be due to long-term compensation for a respiratory acidosis. COPD exacerbations can be infective, however an infective exacerbation would cause the same ABG results but would also cause a fever, raised WCC and raised CRP. Therefore this is likely to be non-infective. Causes of non-infective exacerbations include: non-compliance with medication, exhaustion, mucus plugging and drugs that depress the respiratory centres in the central nervous system such as opiates and benzodiazepines.

All the other answers listed are causes of type 1 respiratory failure. Therefore these would cause hypoxia without a rise in carbon dioxide. It is evident from her baseline ABG that her carbon dioxide levels have increased dramatically and therefore the underlying cause must be something that causes type 2 respiratory failure. The lack of chest pain being reported and gradual onset of symptoms also makes a pneumothorax and pulmonary embolism far less likely.

22. C
Start treatment dose of dalteparin

This patient has a deep vein thrombosis (DVT) in her left calf. Therefore she requires treatment with low molecular weight heparin. She also has a suspected pulmonary embolism (PE) due to her symptoms. The treatment for a DVT and PE are the same, unless it is a massive PE in which case thrombolysis would be required.

Both a computed tomography pulmonary angiogram (CTPA) and ventilation/perfusion scans would be used to confirm the presence of a PE; however the treatment would be the same regardless of whether a PE was present or not. Therefore it is an unnecessary investigation that would expose the unborn child to radiation. In this case neither is required.

Warfarin is teratogenic and therefore not an appropriate form of treatment. This lady would be started on low molecular weight heparin and continue it for at least three months.

23. D
Continuous positive airway pressure (CPAP) and high flow oxygen

This patient has developed acute respiratory distress syndrome (ARDS) as a result of inhalation of fumes. This leads to damage to the airways and causes release of inflammatory mediators, leading to increased capillary permeability and pulmonary oedema. It causes type 1 respiratory failure requiring intensive respiratory support with CPAP and high flow oxygen, to maintain oxygenation of the blood. CPAP is also used in pulmonary oedema and obstructive sleep apnoea.

Twenty-four percent oxygen via a venturi mask is the first level of ventilation used in an exacerbation of chronic obstructive pulmonary disease (COPD). Controlled use of oxygen is used to avoid respiratory depression and carbon dioxide retention. If this is ineffective patients may be trialled on NIPPV and BiPAP, but without giving high concentrations of oxygen. Nebulised salbutamol and 15 L/min of oxygen via a non-rebreath mask would be used in an asthma attack.

24. E
15 litres of oxygen via a non-rebreath mask

This patient has developed carbon monoxide poisoning. This can present non-specifically with a headache, confusion, nausea and vomiting and shortness of breath. On examination the extremities may be pink, because carboxyhaemoglobin appears red in the skin. Pupils may be dilated and ophthalmoscopy may show retinal haemorrhages. Treatment is to give high flow oxygen and transfer to a hyperbaric chamber. This patient had normal oxygen saturations because the sats probe is unable to differentiate between the haemoglobin bound to oxygen and haemoglobin bound to carbon monoxide.

Ceftriaxone is a third generation cephalosporin used to treat meningitis.

Amoxicillin and clarithromycin is a regime used to treat pneumonia.

Naloxone is an antidote for opiate overdose. This would present with constricted pupils, respiratory depression, drowsiness and confusion.

Sodium bicarbonate is given to treat aspirin and tricyclic antidepressant overdoses.

25. D
Unilaterally constricted pupil

This patient has lung cancer, and more specifically has a Pancoast tumour. This is a tumour present in the apex of the lung. It can lead to brachial plexus invasion (causing weakness, pain and paraesthesia), invasion of the recurrent laryngeal nerve (causing dysphonia) and invasion of the sympathetic chain (causing Horner's syndrome which consists of miosis, ptosis, anhidrosis and enophthalmos).

Erythema nodosum is a rash that classically occurs on the shins and forms tender raised purple nodules. It can occur in tuberculosis and sarcoidosis. Other causes include Streptococcal infections, pregnancy, autoimmune conditions such as inflammatory bowel disease and Bechet's disease and drugs such as sulphonamides, the oral contraceptive pill and penicillins.

A new pan-systolic murmur would suggest either mitral or tricuspid regurgitation. This could occur as a result of infective endocarditis and would also present with a fever. Other acute causes would include a myocardial infarction, which has resulted in rupture of the mitral valve papillary muscles.

Haematuria suggests renal/urological pathology. Neither of these is likely in this scenario.

Stridor is caused by upper airway obstruction. This could occur if there was invasion of the trachea by the tumour. Other causes of stridor include laryngeal carcinomas, anaphylaxis, bilateral recurrent laryngeal nerve palsy, infections (epiglottitis, larygnotracheobronchitis/croup) and foreign body inhalation.

26. D
Positive cold direct Coombs test

This patient has been infected with Mycoplasma pneumoniae. It classically occurs in epidemics every few years and presents as an atypical pneumonia with fever, malaise, arthralgia and a dry cough. Atypical pneumonias don't cause lobar consolidation. Instead Mycoplasma causes reticulo-nodular shadowing or patchy consolidation. Due to the absence of a cell wall it cannot be stained and therefore diagnosis is made by serology or polymerase chain reactions (PCR). Complications of a Mycoplasma pneumoniae infection include erythema multiforme (the target shaped rash), which can progress to Stevens-Johnson syndrome, Guillain-Barre syndrome, meningoencephalitis, myelitis and a cold autoimmune haemolytic anaemia. A cold autoimmune haemolytic anaemia is caused by cold agglutinins and would give a positive cold direct Coombs test.

Lobar consolidation is more likely to occur in typical pneumonias, classically caused by Streptococcus pneumoniae (which is the main gram-positive cocci cause of a pneumonia), Haemophilus influenzae, Staphylococcus aureus and Moraxella catarrhalis (which is the main gram-negative cocci cause of pneumonia).

Alpha haemolytic gram-positive diplococcus chains, are describing Streptococcus pneumoniae.

27. B
Streptococcus pneumoniae

Streptococcus pneumoniae (pneumococcus) forms gram-positive diplococcus chains and is alpha-haemolytic (partial haemolysis that causes the agar to turn green). It is the most common cause of pneumonia. Those at a higher risk include the elderly, immunocompromised patients, patients post-splenectomy (because it is an encapsulated organism) and those with heart failure or pre-existing lung disease. It causes a typical pneumonia with lobar consolidation and rust-coloured sputum.

Haemophilus influenza is a gram-negative rod, which also causes a typical pneumonia, but is less common than pneumococcus.

Staphylococcus aureus is a gram-positive coccus that forms clusters when cultured. It also causes a typical pneumonia and classically occurs following an influenza infection. It is a cause of abscess formation that can lead to lung cavities.

Chlamydophilia psittaci causes psittacosis, which is typically acquired from infected birds. It is a cause of an atypical pneumonia.

Influenza is a virus that causes 'the flu' which typically presents with a fever, non-productive cough, muscle and joint aches.

28. D
Sleep studies

This patient has developed obstructive sleep apnoea. This is caused by intermittent closure of the upper airways during sleep. It causes apnoeic episodes and leads to the patient waking up regularly throughout the night. It presents with snoring, daytime somnolence, poor sleep quality and reduced cognitive performance. It can cause type 2 respiratory failure. It is associated with hypertension and obesity. The diagnosis is confirmed by used of sleep studies. These include use of pulse oximetry, video recordings and polysomnography to monitor what occurs during sleep.

Zopiclone belongs to a group called the Z-drugs and is a non-benzodiazepine hypnotic drug. A short course may be prescribed to treat insomnia, but it has no role in obstructive sleep apnoea. It may worsen the condition, as one of its side effects is respiratory depression.

Antidepressants may be used if this patient were thought to have insomnia as a result of a depressive episode, however there is nothing in the history to suggest this.

Neither of the other investigations have a role in diagnosing obstructive sleep apnoea.

29. C
Increased capillary permeability

A para-pneumonic effusion is an exudative effusion that occurs as a result of an underlying pneumonia. The presence of infection leads to increased inflammatory markers, vasodilation and increased capillary permeability.

Decreased oncotic pressure would occur in patients with hypoalbumi-naemia such as in nephrotic syndrome, which causes a transudative effusion.

Impaired lymphatic drainage can occur as a result of lymphangitis, which is inflammation of the lymphatic channels. Lymphangitis carcinoma-tosis is the spread of cancer via the lymphatics. It often leads to obstruction of the lymphatics, which causes interstitial oedema and pleural effusions.

Destruction of the visceral pleura could occur if a peripheral lung cancer was to invade the pleura or as a result of a mesothelioma; both of which would cause exudative pleural effusions.

Elevated hydrostatic pressure can occur as a result of left sided heart failure. There is poor flow through the lungs and a build up of fluid as a result, causing a transudative pleural effusion.

30. C
Erythromycin

This patient has developed theophylline toxicity. Theophylline is an adenosine receptor antagonist and phosphodiesterase inhibitor, which is used as a third line medication to treat both asthma and COPD. It has a narrow therapeutic index and can become toxic quite easily. Precipitants of toxicity include co-prescription of P450 inhibitors such as erythromycin. Toxicity presents with abdominal pain, nausea, vomiting, diarrhoea, and tachycardia. It can lead to arrhythmias and seizures. Blood tests may show hypophosphataemia, hypokalaemia, hypomagnesaemia, hyperglycaemia and a metabolic acidosis.

Rifampicin is a P450 inducer and therefore would reduce theo-phylline levels, rather than causing toxicity. The other drugs listed don't affect the P450 system.

Rheumatology Questions

1. A patient being treated for severe hypertension develops pain in her hands, a malar rash and mouth ulcers. Which of the following drugs is responsible for her symptoms?

A. Doxazosin
B. Hydralazine
C. Indapamide
D. Felodipine
E. Irbesartan

2. A 35-year-old Afro-Caribbean woman presents to clinic with longstanding tightening of the skin on her hands, dysphagia and hard white subcutaneous nodules in her fingertips. She complains of recent bilateral ankle swelling. On examination a parasternal heave is present and a loud P2 can be heard. She has already been prescribed a strong immunosuppressive regime. Which of the following drugs should now be prescribed?

A. Methotrexate
B. Bisoprolol
C. Bosentan
D. Captopril
E. Prednisolone

3. A 22-year-old male presents to hospital with a red, hot, swollen knee. On examination he has an antalgic gait. He has no significant past medical history. The aspirate from the knee is cultured, and grows gram-negative diplococci and the nucleic acid amplification test (NAAT) is positive. Considering the underlying diagnosis how should this patient be treated?

A. Diclofenac
B. Prednisolone
C. Flucloxacillin and fusidic acid
D. Clindamycin
E. Ceftriaxone

4. An elderly lady with longstanding rheumatoid arthritis presents to her doctor with itching in both of her eyes. She describes both eyes as feeling gritty and also describes having a dry mouth. Which of the following is the most likely underlying diagnosis?

A. Allergic conjunctivitis
B. Keratoconjunctivitis sicca
C. Episcleritis
D. Anterior uveitis
E. Blepharitis

5. A young lady presents to her doctor with pain in both of her hands and an erythematous rash on her face and both arms. On examination she has redness and swelling in multiple joints in her hands and multiple mouth ulcers. Her only significant past medical history is an episode of pericarditis diagnosed a few months ago. Which of the following is the most likely diagnosis?

A. Rheumatoid arthritis
B. Systemic lupus erythematosus (SLE)
C. Psoriatic arthritis
D. Systemic sclerosis
E. Polymyositis

6. A 78-year-old retired coal worker presents with dyspnea. On examination it is noted that he has ulnar deviation of the metacarpophalangeal joints and tenderness in the lateral two proximal interphalangeal joints in both hands. His chest X-ray shows multiple bilateral nodules. What is the most likely underlying diagnosis?

A. Pulmonary fibrosis
B. Hypertrophic pulmonary osteoarthropathy
C. Sarcoidosis
D. Caplan's syndrome
E. Felty's syndrome

7. A 28-year-old woman presents to her doctor complaining of recurrent unilateral throbbing headaches, associated with nausea and vomiting. Her past medical history consists of two miscarriages and a deep vein thrombosis. Which of the following findings is most consistent with the underlying diagnosis?

A. Raised platelets
B. Prolonged activated partial thromboplastin time (APTT)
C. Positive anti-Scl-70 antibody
D. Positive anti-Jo1 antibody
E. Antithrombin deficiency

8. A 35-year-old male presents to hospital with a painful red eye. On examination of his eye the pupil appears slightly constricted and irregular in shape. He also reports having a painful genital ulcer and two mouth ulcers. He has a previous history of two deep vein thromboses. Which of the following findings is most consistent with the underlying diagnosis?

A. Human leukocyte antigen B27 (HLA B27)
B. Atypical anti-neutrophil cytoplasmic antibodies (X-ANCA)
C. Perinuclear anti-neutrophil cytoplasmic antibodies (P-ANCA)
D. Positive pathergy test
E. Normal serum c-reactive protein (CRP)

9. A 77-year-old woman presents to her doctor with bilateral shoulder pain. She describes her shoulders feeling stiff and aching in the morning. On examination her shoulders are tender but she has normal power in all of her shoulder movements. Her initial blood tests show a normocytic anaemia, and a raised erythrocyte sedimentation rate and serum c-reactive protein. Which of the following is the most likely diagnosis?

A.   Bilateral osteoarthritis of the shoulders
B.   Rheumatoid arthritis
C.   Polymyositis
D.   Polymyalgia rheumatica (PMR)
E.   Ankylosing spondylitis

10. Which of the following is the most accurate description of rheumatoid factor?

A.   IgM antibody against the alpha chain
B.   IgM antibody against the gamma chain
C.   IgM antibody against the kappa chain
D.   IgG antibody against the alpha chain
E.   IgG antibody against the delta chain

11. A 25-year-old male presents to clinic with lower back pain. He describes his back as feeling stiff in the morning, and says the stiffness is relieved by exercise. On examination he has tenderness of the sacroiliac joints. Which of the following findings is most consistent with the underlying diagnosis?

A.   Normal forced expiratory volume in one second / forced vital capacity (FEV$_1$/FVC) ratio
B.   Positive rheumatoid factor
C.   Positive Schirmer's test
D.   Symmetrical small joint polyarthritis
E.   Macrocytic anaemia

12. A 78-year-old Caucasian male presents to clinic with deep boring bone pain in his leg. On examination it is noticed he has bowing of his tibia and new onset sensorineural deafness in his left ear. Routine bloods and an X-ray of his tibia are taken. Considering the underlying diagnosis what is the most likely finding in this patient's investigations?

A. Normal X-ray
B. Looser's zones on the X-ray
C. Cortical thickening and sclerosis on the X-ray
D. Hypercalcaemia
E. Hypocalcaemia

13. A 23-year-old female presents to hospital with haematuria. On examination it is noticed she has a malar rash on her face and mouth ulcers. A urine dip shows blood +++ and protein +++. What medication should this patient be started on?

A. Azathioprine
B. Methotrexate
C. Hydroxychloroquine
D. Prednisolone and cyclophosphamide
E. Sulfasalazine

14. A patient presents to hospital with severe central crushing chest pain. On examination an ulcerating vasculitic rash was noticed on his skin. When an angiography was performed it was noticed he has multiple aneurysms in the coronary arteries. His only significant past medical history is renal impairment, and a previous renal angiogram also showed multiple aneurysms. Which of the following findings is most consistent with the underlying diagnosis?

A. Cytoplasmic anti-neutrophil cytoplasmic antibodies (C-ANCA)
B. Raised serum C3
C. Hepatitis B surface antibody positive
D. Hepatitis B surface antigen positive
E. Detection of hepatitis C RNA by polymerase chain reaction (PCR)

15. A 34-year-old pregnant woman with known systemic lupus erythe-matosus (SLE) is on the labour ward. On giving birth her child is brady-cardic, and an electrocardiogram (ECG) shows third degree heart block. Which of the following is the underlying cause of her child's bradycardia?

A. Treatment with hydroxychloroquine
B. Treatment with rituximab
C. Anti-Sm antibody
D. Anti-Ro antibody
E. Anti-La antibody

16. A 40-year-old Caucasian woman presents to clinic with pain in both of her hands. She describes having morning stiffness in the small joints in both hands. On examination she has bilateral ulnar deviation, and swelling and tenderness of the small joints in her hands, with Boutonniere's deformity in the index fingers of both hands. A full autoimmune screen is requested. Which of the follow-ing is most specific for the underlying diagnosis?

A. Anti-cyclic citrullinated peptide (anti-CCP) antibody
B. Antinuclear antibodies (ANA)
C. Rheumatoid factor
D. Anti-Sm antibody
E. Anti-centromere antibody

17. A patient presents to clinic with increasing fatigue and weakness. She also described developing a rash whenever she was exposed to the sun. On exami-nation her proximal muscles appear weak and are tender to touch. Roughened red papules can be seen over the knuckles of both hands. A chest X-ray shows areas of pulmonary fibrosis. Considering the underlying diagnosis, which of the following antibodies is linked with pulmonary fibrosis in this patient?

A. Rheumatoid factor
B. Anti-Jo1
C. Anti-Mi2
D. Anti-RNP
E. Anti-dsDNA

9"x6"   b3668   320 Single Best Answer Questions for Final Year Medical Students
b3668_03-Gastrointestinal.indd   93   23-Aug-19 6:

Rheumatology Questions   281

18. A patient presents to a rheumatology clinic with pain in both her hands. An antibody screen shows the following:

Antinuclear antibodies (ANA):	positive
Anti-Ro antibody:	positive
Anti-La antibody:	positive
Anti-cyclic citrullinated peptide (CCP) antibody:	negative
Anti-double stranded DNA (dsDNA) antibody:	positive
Rheumatoid factor:	positive

What is the most likely underlying diagnosis?

A. Systemic lupus erythematosus (SLE)
B. Rheumatoid arthritis
C. Sjogren's syndrome
D. Systemic sclerosis
E. Psoriatic arthritis

19. A 24-year-old male presents to clinic with jaundice. As he enters the clinic the doctor notices he has a forward stopping posture and a loss of arm swing. He is slow to sit down and when he does it is clear that he has a unilateral resting tremor. On taking a full history he also reports having pain in some of his joints. As a result an X-ray of his left knee is requested. Considering the underlying diagnosis what is the most likely finding on the X-ray?

A. Subchondral sclerosis
B. Juxta-articular osteopenia
C. Looser's zones
D. Chondrocalcinosis
E. Periarticular erosions

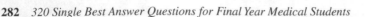

20. A patient presents to his doctor with his concerned wife. His wife has been complaining that he has been making loud breathing noises during his sleep. On examination he is found to have a saddle shaped nose and the doctor also notices his pinna are more mobile than normal, giving the appearance of floppy ears. What is the most likely underlying diagnosis?

A. Granulomatosis with polyangiitis
B. Mixed connective tissue disease
C. Relapsing polychondritis
D. Marfan syndrome
E. Cocaine abuse

21. A 60-year-old male with a history of alcoholism, hypertension, type 2 diabetes mellitus and obesity is started on indapamide to control his blood pressure. Two weeks later he presents to hospital with a red, hot swollen left wrist. He is apyrexial. A joint aspirate is performed. Which of the following is most likely to be seen on microscopy and serology?

A. Rhomboid shaped crystals with weakly positive birefringence
B. Needle shaped crystals with strongly negative birefringence
C. Gram-positive clusters of diplococci
D. Giant cells
E. Immune complexes formed by large IgM proteins

22. A patient taking methotrexate to control rheumatoid arthritis presents to her doctor with a fever, and is due to be prescribed antibiotics. Which of the following antibiotics is contraindicated in this patient?

A. Metronidazole
B. Trimethoprim
C. Clindamycin
D. Vancomycin
E. Isoniazid

23. A 45-year-old lady with brittle asthma presents to her doctor with a dull back pain in the thoracic region. She states that it has come on gradually and improves when she lies down, but is worse after standing and walking around. On examination she is found to have a slumped posture and appears to have lost some height since her last appointment, but not experienced any weight loss. Which of the following is the most likely diagnosis?

A. Spinal metastases
B. Spinal osteoarthritis
C. Spinal crush fracture
D. Ankylosing spondylitis
E. Paget's disease

24. A 23-year-old female who is taking the combined oral contraceptive pill is prescribed lymecycline to treat her acne. Subsequently she develops pain in her hands, mouth ulcers and a rash on her skin when she uses sun beds. Which of the following is most likely to be positive in this patient?

A. Anti-dsDNA antibodies
B. Anti-histone antibodies
C. Anti-Jo1 antibodies
D. Anti-cardiolipin antibodies
E. Anti-centromere antibodies

25. A 75-year-old lady presents with a painful throbbing temporal headache, which is made worse by brushing her hair. She is also experiencing jaw claudication. Her blood tests show a normocytic normochromic anaemia, and raised erythrocyte sedimentation rate (ESR). Which of the following should occur next?

A. Commence high dose prednisolone
B. Temporal artery biopsy
C. Computed tomography (CT) scan of her head
D. Administer ibuprofen and sumatriptan
E. Start high flow oxygen

26. A tall male patient is referred to a rheumatologist to investigate his recurrent back pain. On examination he is found to have a large arm-span, high arched palate and scoliosis. His past medical history includes recurrent pneumothoracies and aortic dissection. Which of the following is responsible for his symptoms?

A. Autosomal dominant mutation in the vHL tumour suppressor gene
B. Autosomal dominant mutation in the fibrillin gene
C. Autosomal dominant mutation in the collagen gene
D. X-linked recessive mutation in the collagen type IV gene
E. Overexpression of the IGF-2 gene

27. A 65-year-old lady with a history of alcoholic liver cirrhosis presents to her doctor with pain in her knee. She states that it has gradually worsened over the past year, and is always worse by the end of the day. On examination her knee feels boggy and there is a positive patella tap. She is found to have a reduced range of movement and crepitus can be felt on passive movement of the knee. Which of the following is the most appropriate first line treatment of her condition?

A. Paracetamol
B. Glucosamine sulfate
C. Codeine phosphate
D. Naproxen
E. Total knee replacement

28. A patient is prescribed long-term high dose prednisolone by her rheumatologist. Which of the following combinations of medications should also be started?

A. Alfacalcidol and calcium supplements
B. Captopril and metformin
C. Raloxifene and ranitidine
D. Alendronic acid and lanzoprazole
E. Magnesium trisilicate and gliclazide

29. A 30-year-old lady presents with pain in both her hands. On examination she has pain and swelling in the distal interphalangeal joints of all four fingers on both hands. Plain radiographs of both hands are requested and show a 'pencil in cup' deformity at the affected joints. Which of the following is the most likely underlying diagnosis?

A. Osteoarthritis
B. Rheumatoid arthritis
C. Systemic lupus erythematosus (SLE)
D. Enteropathic arthropathy
E. Psoriatic arthritis

30. A 40-year-old man presents with sudden onset back pain which started two days ago. He describes the pain as sharp, and it radiates down his right leg. It can be reproduced if he lies down and elevates his leg to 20 degrees. Which of the following findings would be most consistent with the underlying diagnosis?

A. Perianal anaesthesia
B. Loss of sensation on the dorsal lateral aspect of the foot
C. Upward going plantars
D. Urinary retention
E. Erosive changes seen on an X-ray of the lumbar spine

Rheumatology Answers

1. B
Hydralazine

This woman has developed drug-induced lupus. Many different drugs can cause this; but those well known for causing it are hydralazine, isoniazid, quinidine, procainamide, tetracycline antibiotics and phenytoin. Drug induced lupus is associated with anti-histone antibodies. The disease remits once the drug is stopped.

Doxazosin is an alpha-adrenoceptor blocker used as a third line anti-hypertensive and to treat benign prostatic hyperplasia. Its side effects include postural hypotension, incontinence, dry mouth and nasal stuffiness.

Indapamide is a thiazide-like diuretic. Its side effects include electro-lyte imbalances (such as low sodium, low potassium, raised calcium and raised urate) and it can cause impotence in men.

Felodipine is a dihydropyridine calcium channel blocker. Its side effects include headache, ankle swelling, facial flushing, reflex tachycardia and gum hypertrophy.

Irbesartan is an angiotensin II receptor blocker. Side effects include hyperkalaemia and acute kidney injury.

2. C
Bosentan

This woman has developed pulmonary hypertension as a result of her underlying limited systemic sclerosis. This should be treated with bosentan, which is an endothelin 1 receptor antagonist and a vasodilator of the pulmonary arteries. Sildenafil is a phosphodiesterase inhibitor that can also be used to treat pulmonary hypertension.

Limited systemic sclerosis presents with CREST syndrome (subcutaneous calcification, Raynaud's phenomenon, oesophageal dysmotility, sclerodactyly and telangiectasia). It also causes tightening of the skin, which is limited to the hands, forearms, feet and face. Signs of pulmonary hypertension include a loud P2, parasternal heave, hepatomegaly and ankle swelling.

Captopril is an angiotensin converting enzyme (ACE) inhibitor that is often used in heart failure, and would also be prescribed in systemic sclerosis with renal involvement to prevent a renal crisis. Bisoprolol is a beta-blocker and can be used to treat heart failure, but would not treat the underlying pulmonary hypertension.

Methotrexate and prednisolone would both be used as a form of immunosuppression. Steroids should be avoided in systemic sclerosis as they can precipitate a renal crisis. The most commonly used immunosuppressive agents are cyclophosphamide and mycophenolate mofetil.

3. E
Ceftriaxone

This patient has developed septic arthritis. This presents with a red, hot, swollen joint and a fever. The most common cause of septic arthritis is Staphylococcus aureus, which is a gram-positive coccus. However the most common cause in young adults is Neisseria gonorrhoeae. It is a gram-negative diplococcus, which can also be tested for by use of NAATs. Ceftriaxone (a third generation cephalosporin) is the most effective antibiotic to treat gonococcal arthritis.

If Staphylococcus aureus were grown in the culture the most effective antibiotic regime would be flucloxacillin and fusidic acid. If a patient is allergic to penicillin then glycopeptide antibiotics such as vancomycin and teicoplanin or clindamycin can be used.

Diclofenac is a non-steroidal anti-inflammatory drug (NSAID) that can be used to treat an acute flare of gout.

Prednisolone is a corticosteroid that can be used to treat a number of autoimmune joint conditions.

4. B
Keratoconjunctivitis sicca

This lady has developed secondary Sjogren's syndrome. This can occur secondary to chronic inflammatory conditions such as rheumatoid arthritis and systemic sclerosis. It is caused by the lymphocytic infiltration and fibrosis of the exocrine glands (especially the lacrimal and salivary glands). It causes reduced production of tears, which causes dry eyes and keratoconjunctivitis sicca, and reduced production of saliva, which causes a dry mouth and xerostomia. It can also cause vaginal dryness, which leads to dyspareunia. The treatment of keratoconjunctivitis sicca is to prescribe artificial tears such as hypromellose eye drops. Pilocarpine is a muscarinic receptor agonist and can be prescribed to increase the production of tears and saliva.

Episcleritis and scleritis can also occur in rheumatoid arthritis but both present with a red eye. Episcleritis is often painless whereas scleritis is extremely painful. In episcleritis the blood vessels will blanch on use of phenylephrine eye drops, whereas in scleritis they will not.

Anterior uveitis presents with a painful red eye, photophobia and an irregularly constricted pupil. On examination with a slit lamp a hypopyon can be seen. It is associated with multiple autoimmune conditions such as ankylosing spondylitis, Bechet's disease, granulomatosis with polyangiitis and sarcoidosis.

Blepharitis causes red, swollen, itchy eyelids. It presents with a gritty feeling in the eyes, and flakes around the roots of the eyelashes. It is treated by regularly washing the eyelids.

Allergic conjunctivitis presents with bilateral itchy eyes, lacrimation and rhinorrhea. Common triggers include household dust, pollen and mold spores.

5. B
Systemic lupus erythematosus (SLE)

This lady has presented with multiple features consistent with SLE. These include a photosensitive rash, arthralgia, mouth ulcers and pericarditis. SLE is an autoimmune multi-system disease caused by autoantibodies against a variety of autoantigens. Other features include a malar rash, discoid rash, serositis such as pleurisy and peritonitis, renal failure, central nervous system disorders such as seizures and psychosis, haematological disorders such as a haemolytic anaemia, leucopenia and thrombocytopenia. The diagnosis is confirmed by testing for autoantibodies such as anti-nuclear antibodies (ANA), anti-double stranded DNA (anti-dsDNA) antibody and anti-Sm antibody.

Rheumatoid arthritis is can also present with a small joint polyarthritis, but is less likely to cause mouth ulcers and pericarditis. Also it doesn't cause a photosensitive rash.

Psoriatic arthritis can present with a small joint arthritis but the rash described would be more classical of a psoriatic rash. This would classically occur on the extensor surfaces and be a salmon pink colour with grey/silvery scales.

Systemic sclerosis would present with skin tightening. If it is limited systemic sclerosis it could cause skin tightening on the hands, forearms, feet and face. Whereas diffuse systemic sclerosis would affect the skin all over the body. Other features include pulmonary fibrosis, pulmonary hypertension, Raynaud's phenomenon, skin calcinosis, arthralgia, dysphagia, and renal crisis that can cause malignant hypertension.

Polymyositis presents with pain and weakness in the proximal muscles such as the deltoids and quadriceps. It is often a paraneoplastic syndrome and once the diagnosis is made patients require extensive screening for an underlying malignancy. The condition responds well to corticosteroids.

6. D
Caplan's syndrome

Caplan's syndrome is a combination of pneumoconiosis and rheumatoid arthritis that coal workers can develop, due to an inflammatory response to external allergens. Smoking is also thought to aggravate Caplan's syndrome. It presents with a cough, shortness of breath, joint pains and swelling and morning stiffness. A chest X-ray would show multiple lung nodules. This patient also has the classic joint pathology associated with rheumatoid arthritis such as ulnar deviation and a symmetrical small joint polyarthritis. The distal interphalangeal joints have been spared.

Felty's syndrome can occur in rheumatoid arthritis and consists of rheumatoid arthritis, neutropenia and splenomegaly.

Pulmonary fibrosis can occur in rheumatoid arthritis but the chest X-ray would show reticulo-nodular shadowing, rather than well-circumscribed lesions.

Sarcoidosis is a multi-system condition that primarily affects the lungs causing bilateral hilar lymphadenopathy and pulmonary fibrosis. It can progress to honeycombing. It also causes arthralgia and terminal phalangeal cysts. Other features include keratoconjunctivitis sicca, xerostomia, uveitis, erythema nodosum, parotid and lacrimal gland enlargement. Complications include hypercalcaemia, facial nerve palsy, meningoencephalitis and cardiomyopathy.

Hypertrophic pulmonary osteoarthropathy is a paraneoplastic syndrome that can occur in lung cancer. It causes painful clubbing of the fingers and toes. There is also distal expansion of the long bones causing pain in the wrists and ankles. It doesn't cause rheumatoid deformities, and a primary lung cancer is more likely to cause a solitary lesion on a chest X-ray rather than multiple bilateral lesions.

9"x6"   b3668   320 Single Best Answer Questions for Final Year Medical Students
b3668_03-Gastrointestinal.indd   103
23-Aug-19 6:

7. B
Prolonged activated partial thromboplastin time (APTT)

This woman has antiphospholipid syndrome. This presents with recurrent arterial and venous thromboses. Other features include migranes, mitral valve prolapse, livedo reticularis, recurrent miscarriages and thrombocytopenia. It is also associated with systemic lupus erythematosus (SLE).

Despite this disease having pro-coagulant affects in-vivo, in-vitro the APTT is prolonged, due to the effect of the lupus anticoagulant antibody in the test tube. Other antibodies found in antiphospholipid syndrome include anti-cardiolipin antibody and anti-beta-2-glycoprotein-1 antibody.

Anti-Scl-70 occurs in diffuse systemic sclerosis and anti-Jo1 in polymyositis and dermatomyositis.

Antithrombin deficiency is a thrombophilia that would cause recurrent venous thromboses. However it is a separate condition to antiphospholipid syndrome.

8. D
Positive pathergy test

This patient has developed Bechet's disease, which is a medium vessel vasculitis. It is characterised by anterior and posterior uveitis, oral and genital ulceration, colitis and both arterial and venous thromboses. In this scenario this patient has anterior uveitis and also both mouth and genital ulcers. The diagnosis is made by a positive pathergy test, which is where a needle prick leads to papule formation.

HLA B27 is associated with seronegative arthritidies, such as ankylosing spondylitis, enteropathic arthritis, psoriatic arthritis and reactive arthritis.

X-ANCA is associated with ulcerative colitis.

P-ANCA can be found in various conditions including ulcerative colitis, eosinophilic granulomatosis with polyangiitis and microscopic polyangiitis.

Most inflammatory conditions would cause a raised CRP. Systemic lupus erythematosus (SLE) classically causes a raised erythrocyte sedimentation rate (ESR) with a normal CRP. This can help differentiate SLE from other autoimmune diseases.

9. D
Polymyalgia rheumatica (PMR)

Polymyalgia rheumatica (PMR) is a chronic inflammatory condition that is closely associated with giant cell arteritis (GCA). It presents with aching, tenderness and morning stiffness in the proximal muscles. However it doesn't cause weakness. It can also cause fevers, weight loss, anorexia and fatigue. Initial blood tests would demonstrate anaemia of chronic disease and raised inflammatory markers. The serum creatine kinase is normal in PMR, which can help differentiate it from a myositis. PMR is treated with a prolonged course of corticosteroids.

Polymyositis would present with pain, and weakness in the proximal muscles, and would also cause a raised serum creatine kinase and raised inflammatory markers. The main reason this patient is unlikely to have polymyositis is because her shoulder muscles are not weak.

Rheumatoid arthritis classically affects the small joints in the hands and feet, and would be unlikely to present for the first time in a patient of this age. The peak onset of rheumatoid arthritis is in the 4th decade of life.

Ankylosing spondylitis is a seronegative arthropathy that presents with back pain and stiffness, which is worse in the morning. It often starts with a sacroiliitis, and therefore the sacroiliac joints can be tender on examination. Ankylosing spondylitis is far more common in men and occurs at a much younger age. Other features include enthesitis, anterior uveitis, aortic valve regurgitation, apical pulmonary fibrosis and amyloidosis.

Bilateral osteoarthritis of the shoulders would cause pain that worsens throughout the day, and gets worse rather than better with movement. Furthermore this patient has raised inflammatory markers indicating that there is a systemic inflammatory condition underlying her presentation. In osteoarthritis there is no systemic inflammation and therefore the inflammatory markers would be normal.

10. B
IgM antibody against the gamma chain

Rheumatoid factor is an antibody against the Fc portion of the gamma chain found in IgG. Most commonly it is of the IgM isotype but it can be formed from any of the other immunoglobulin isotypes.

11. A
Normal forced expiratory volume in one second/forced vital capacity (FEV$_1$/FVC) ratio

This patient has ankylosing spondylitis. This is a seronegative spondyloarthritis, which leads to sacroiliitis and stiffness of the spine. Complications include apical lung fibrosis, which would cause a restrictive pattern in the lung function tests (normal FEV$_1$/FVC ratio, and reduced FEV$_1$). It is worsened by the loss of thoracic spinal movement causing reduced chest expansion. It can also cause a normocytic normochromic anaemia (anaemia of chronic disease) anterior uveitis, amyloidosis, aortic regurgitation, Achilles tendonitis (and other forms of enthesitis), osteoporosis and an asymmetrical large joint oligoarthritis (rather than a symmetrical small joint polyarthritis that is found in rheumatoid arthritis and systemic lupus erythematosus [SLE]).

The seronegative spondyloarthritides test negative for rheumatoid factor.

Schirmer's test is used to diagnose keratoconjunctivitis sicca, which occurs in Sjogren's syndrome. It involves putting a strip of filter paper under the lower eyelid and measuring the distance that the tears travel. If it is <5 mm in 5 minutes the test is positive.

12. C
Cortical thickening and sclerosis on the X-ray

This patient has Paget's disease, which is an idiopathic remodelling of the bone caused by increased bone turnover and increased activity of both osteoblasts and osteoclasts. This leads to bone enlargement, deformities and pathological fractures. Other complications include sensorineural deafness due to remodelling of the petrosal bone causing compression of the vestibulocochlear nerve, osteoarthritis, high output congestive cardiac failure and osteosarcoma. Hypercalcaemia can occur but only if the patient is immobile. The most common blood findings are a normal serum calcium and serum phosphate but a raised alkaline phosphatase (ALP). The X-ray of the tibia is likely to show a saber tibia, which consists of a bowing deformity, patchy cortical thickening and sclerosis.

Looser's zones are found in osteomalacia and these are where there are apparent fractures, without displacement.

13. D
Prednisolone and cyclophosphamide

This patient has developed systemic lupus erythematosus (SLE) nephritis and requires high dose steroids and cyclophosphamide for immunosuppression. Oral prednisolone is preferred to hydrocortisone because it is stronger. Cyclophosphamide should be given with MESNA to prevent haemorrhagic cystitis.

Hydroxychloroquine and methotrexate can be used to maintain remission. Hydroxychloroquine is often first line, and immunosuppressants, such as methotrexate and azathioprine, are only used in severe disease.

14. D
Hepatitis B surface antigen positive

This patient has polyarteritis nodosa. This is an anti-neutrophil cyto-plasmic antibodies (ANCA) negative medium vessel vasculitis, which affects the heart and kidneys. It is associated with a hepatitis B virus infection. Hepatitis B surface antigen is a marker of current infection, whereas hepatitis B surface antibody is a marker of immu-nity to the hepatitis B virus. Other features of polyarteritis nodosa are abdominal pain, polyarthralgia, vasculitic rash, multiple skin ulcers, mononeuritis multiplex and sensory polyneuropathy.

In inflammatory states C3 and C4 levels decrease and there is increased C3d and C4d, due to increased compliment activity. There is also likely to be raised serum c-reactive protein (CRP) and eryth-rocyte sedimentation rate (ESR) levels.

15. D
Anti-Ro antibody

The anti-Ro antibody is able to cross the placenta and can result in com-plete heart block in the neonate. Anti-Ro can be found in both systemic lupus erythematosus (SLE) and Sjogren's syndrome. Anti-La is another antibody that can be found in both these conditions, however anti-La is unable to cross the placenta. Anti-Sm is the most specific antibody for SLE, and doesn't cross the placenta.

Hydroxychloroquine is regarded as safe during pregnancy. Its side effects include retinopathy and lowering the seizure threshold. Rituximab is not regarded as safe in pregnancy, but doesn't cause complete heart block.

16. A
Anti-cyclic citrullinated peptide (anti-CCP) antibody

This lady has an underlying diagnosis of rheumatoid arthritis. This is evident because of the small joint, symmetrical polyarthritis that has been described. Furthermore she has developed Boutonniere's deformity, which describes proximal interphalangeal (PIP) joint flex-ion with distal interphalangeal (DIP) joint hyperextension, and this can occur in poorly controlled rheumatoid arthritis. Other deformities that can occur in long-standing in rheumatoid arthritis include ulnar deviation, swan neck deformities of the fingers and Z-deformities of the thumbs. Anti-cyclic citrullinated peptide (anti-CCP) antibody is the most specific test for diagnosing rheumatoid arthritis.

Rheumatoid factor is positive in 70% of patients with rheuma-toid arthritis, but can also be positive in many other conditions. Rheumatoid factor is positive in nearly 100% of patients with Sjogren's syndrome and Felty's syndrome, and is positive in a minority of patients with systemic lupus erythematosus (SLE) and systemic sclerosis.

Antinuclear antibodies (ANA) are positive in about 30% of patients with rheumatoid arthritis, but is a more sensitive and specific test for diagnosing SLE and is present in 90% of patients with SLE.

Anti-Sm antibody is a highly specific test for diagnosing SLE, but has a poor sensitivity, as it is only present in a minority of patients.

Anti-centromere antibody is specific to limited systemic sclerosis.

17. B
Anti-Jo1

This patient has dermatomyositis and has presented with proximal muscle weakness and tenderness, a photosensitive rash and Gottron's papules on the hands. These are red roughened papules over the knuckles. The com-bination of Gottron's papules, muscle weakness and a raised creatine kinase (CK) is pathognomonic of dermatomyositis.

This patient has developed anti-synthetase syndrome, a cause of dermatomyositis and polymyositis, which occurs as a result of autoantibodies formed against aminoacyl-tRNA synthetases. The most common of these antibodies is anti-Jo1. Features of anti-synthetase syndrome include interstitial lung disease, inflammatory myopathy, small joint polyarthritis, Raynaud's phenomenon and mechanic's hands (painful rough fissuring of the skin on the finger tips and lateral aspects of the fingers).

Other cutaneous features of dermatomyositis include shawl sign (a macular photosensitive rash over the back and shoulders), heliotrope rash (a lilac-purple rash on the eyelids), subcutaneous calcifications and dilated capillary loops in the nail folds.

Both dermatomyositis and polymyositis are associated with anti-Jo1 and anti-Mi2 antibodies. However only anti-Jo1 antibodies have a strong association with pulmonary fibrosis, due to the development of anti-synthetase syndrome.

Anti-RNP antibody is found in both mixed connective tissue disease and systemic lupus erythematosus (SLE). Anti-dsDNA antibody is found in SLE. Rheumatoid factor is found in a lot of conditions. It is found in almost all people with Sjogren's syndrome and Felty's syndrome. It can be found in rheumatoid arthritis but is not very sensitive or specific, but if positive it may indicate patients are more likely to develop extra-articular complications. Other conditions that may test positive for rheumatoid factor are infections (infective endocarditis, hepatitis), SLE and systemic sclerosis. It is also a normal finding in a small proportion of the population.

18. C
Sjogren's syndrome

Rheumatoid factor is present in almost 100% of patients with Sjogren's syndrome. Anti-Ro and anti-La antibodies are also found in Sjogren's syndrome. Anti-dsDNA antibody is negative, which makes SLE less likely. The presence of rheumatoid factor means it is unlikely to be psoriatic arthritis, as it is seronegative. Although rheumatoid arthritis can cause a positive rheumatoid factor, it wouldn't cause both anti-Ro and anti-La antibodies to be produced. Furthermore the anti-CCP antibody is negative, making rheumatoid arthritis very unlikely in this case.

19. D
Chondrocalcinosis

This patient has Wilson's syndrome, which is caused by an autosomal recessive mutation in the copper transporting ATPase. This leads to copper deposition in the liver (causing liver cirrhosis) and basal ganglia (resulting in parkinsonism). It also causes arthralgia due to pseudogout, which presents with chondrocalcinosis. Other features of Wilson's disease include dementia, psychosis, ataxia, dystonias and dysarthria. Signs include Kayser-Fleischer rings and blue lunulae.

Other causes of pseudogout include diabetes mellitus, hyperparathyroidism, hypothyroidism, hereditary haemochromatosis, hypomagnesaemia and hypophosphataemia. It is caused by deposition of rhomboid shaped calcium pyrophosphate crystals, which have a weakly positive birefringence, in the joints.

Subchondral sclerosis occurs in osteoarthritis. Other radiological changes that occur in osteoarthritis include subchondral cysts, loss of joint space and osteophytes.

Juxta-articular osteopenia occurs in rheumatoid arthritis. Other radiological changes that occur in rheumatoid arthritis are loss of joint space, soft tissue swelling and joint deformities (such as subluxation, hyperextension and ulnar deviation).

Looser's zones occur in osteomalacia, and these are where there are apparent fractures, without displacement.

Periarticular erosions occur in both gout and rheumatoid arthritis and can lead to deformities.

20. C
Relapsing polychondritis

Relapsing polychondritis is a multi-system autoimmune disease caused by inflammation and destruction of cartilage. The breakdown and loss of cartilage affects the ears causing floppy, cauliflower ears. Destruction of the nasal septum causes a saddle shaped nose. Destruction of the laryngeal and tracheal cartilage leads to the patient's upper airways becoming blocked and causes stridor. This is the loud noise this patient is making when he is asleep. Involvement of the ribs causes costochondritis and involvement of the joints causes arthritis.

Granulomatosis with polyangiitis, formerly known as Wegener's granulomatosis, is a small vessel cytoplasmic anti-neutrophil cytoplasmic antibodies (C-ANCA) positive vasculitis. It affects the lungs, kidneys, eyes and upper airways. It can also cause destruction of the nasal septum and a saddle shaped nose, but it doesn't affect the ears.

Mixed connective tissue disease often presents as a combination of a few connective tissue diseases such as systemic sclerosis, systemic lupus erythematosus (SLE) and polymyositis. It may test positive for anti-RNP antibody. This condition often doesn't fall into the diagnostic criteria for just one of the autoimmune conditions.

Marfan syndrome is caused by an autosomal dominant mutation in the fibrillin gene in chromosome 15. This can be inherited or sporadic. It causes arachnodactyly, high arched palate, wide arm-span, scoliosis and pes planus. Complications include upwards lens dislocation, aortic valve regurgitation, aortic dissection and pneumothorax.

Cocaine abuse can also cause destruction of the nasal septum and a saddle shaped nose. Patients may have recurrent epistaxis, perforated septum, snoring due to nasal collapse and anosmia. It has detrimental effects on the heart, which include tachycardia, arrhythmias, aortic dissection, coronary artery vasospasm and myocardial infarction. Other systemic affects include weight loss, insomnia, anxiety and addiction.

21. B
Needle shaped crystals with strongly negative birefringence

This patient is most likely to have gout. The reason for this is because he has multiple risk factors. Hypertension, obesity and insulin resistance all are suggestive of metabolic syndrome, which is linked with gout. Secondly alcohol is likely to increase his purine levels and thus put him at a higher risk of gout, and finally he was recently started on indapamide, which is a thiazide-like diuretic. Both thiazide and loop diuretics are known to increase the uric acid levels in the blood.

Other drugs that can do so are pyrazinamide and chemotherapy/cytotoxic drugs. The indapamide is likely to have triggered this attack. Needle shaped crystals with strongly negative birefringence are found in gout.

Rhomboid shaped crystals with weakly positive birefringence are found in pseudogout.

Gram-positive clusters of diplococci would most likely be Staphylococcus aureus, a cause of septic arthritis. This is less likely as the patient is apyrexial.

Giant cells are formed from macrophages and are found in granulomas.

Immune complexes formed by large IgM proteins are suggestive of rheumatoid factor. There is no suggestion of multiple joint involvement or extra-articular features, so this is unlikely.

22. B
Trimethoprim

Trimethoprim acts by binding to and inhibiting bacterial dihydro-folate reductase. This inhibits the reduction of dihydrofolic acid and prevents DNA synthesis.

Methotrexate acts by competitively inhibiting human dihydro-folate reductase. It is thought that if these drugs were co-prescribed they would lead to a severe folate deficiency.

If isoniazid and methotrexate are co-prescribed it can lead to an increased risk of hepatotoxicity. However this is not a complete contraindication. It just requires strict monitoring of liver function tests.

23. C
Spinal crush facture

Spinal crush fractures can present acutely or be relatively asymptomatic for a period of time. They occur as a result of osteoporosis. Despite this patient being young she also has brittle asthma and therefore is likely to have received lots of courses of steroids in the past. This would hasten the onset of osteoporosis. Spinal crush fractures should be suspected in anyone who has lost height. They also cause pain that is worse on movement and better at rest.

Spinal metastases could occur as a result of breast, lung, thyroid, kidney or prostate cancer. They would cause weight loss, nocturnal pain, fevers and night sweats, and also could cause symptoms of hypercalcaemia. This patient has no history of malignancy and no weight loss, making this unlikely. However spinal metastases can lead to pathological spinal fractures.

Osteoarthritis would be unlikely at this age and doesn't commonly affect the spinal joints. It is more likely to affect the hip or the knee. Also it wouldn't cause a loss of height.

Ankylosing spondylitis is an autoimmune condition affecting the spine. It often starts in the sacroiliac joints and causes morning stiffness, which would improve upon exercise. It is more likely to affect young men. It can cause a loss of height, but this would be after severe progression of the condition and formation of what is known as a bamboo spine. This loss of height would be due to the patient not being able to stand up straight, rather than their spine shortening in length.

Paget's disease is an idiopathic condition that causes remodelling of the bone. It more commonly affects middle-aged/old men and is rare in patients under the age of 40 years old. Common sites include the tibia and petrosal bone. The pain is described as a deep boring pain, and there is often deformation of the bone. Complications can include fractures, nerve compression, high output cardiac failure, osteosarcoma, osteoarthritis and hypercalcaemia if the patient is immobile.

24. B
Anti-histone antibodies

This patient has developed drug induced lupus; which presents with features of systemic lupus erythematosus (SLE) such as small joint polyarthralgia, mouth ulcers, alopecia, malar rash and photosensitive rash. It is caused by anti-histone antibodies and often the disease remits once the drug is stopped. Other causes of drug induced lupus include hydralazine, any tetracycline antibiotic (such as lymecyline, minocycline, and doxycyline), procainamide, quinidine, chlorprom-azine, phenytoin, isoniazid and sulphasalazine.

Anti-dsDNA antibodies are found in SLE, but not in drug induced lupus.

Anti-Jo1 is found in both polymyositis and dermatomyositis and is specific to a subtype of these conditions known as anti-synthetase syndrome.

Anti-cardiolipin antibodies are found in anti-phospholipid syn-drome, but are not very specific. They can also be positive in SLE, pregnancy, immunisation, pneumonia, syphilis, malaria, tuberculosis and leprosy infections.

Anti-centromere antibodies are found in limited systemic sclerosis.

25. A
Commence high dose prednisolone

This patient has developed giant cell arteritis (GCA); which is a large ves-sel vasculitis caused by granulomatous inflammation. A biopsy would show giant cells infiltrating the tissue, and is the gold standard for diagno-sis. However GCA can cause skip lesions and therefore a biopsy may miss the affected area, giving a false negative result. If a diagnosis is suspected then high dose prednisolone must be started immediately. GCA can lead to irreversible blindness if left untreated, and therefore is an emergency.

It presents with a temporal headache, scalp tenderness, jaw claudication and amaurosis fugax. It is also associated with polymyalgia rheumatica, which causes proximal muscle aches, tenderness and morning stiffness. Blood tests classically show an extremely high erythrocyte sedimentation rate (ESR), raised serum c-reactive protein (CRP), normocytic normochromic anaemia, raised platelets and raised alkaline phosphatase (ALP).

Temporal artery biopsy would confirm the diagnosis, but treatment should be initiated first.

A computed tomography (CT) scan of the head may be used if a patient was suspected to have a space-occupying lesion or a history of trauma.

Ibuprofen and sumatriptan are used to treat migraines, which would present with a unilateral throbbing headache, nausea and vomiting, photophobia and phonophobia and may be preceded by a visual aura.

High flow oxygen is used to treat a cluster headache, which would present with a severe, unilateral headache with pain often localised around the eye. This is accompanied by autonomic symptoms such as lacrimation and rhinorrhea.

26. B
Autosomal dominant mutation in the fibrillin gene

This patient has Marfan syndrome, which is caused by an autosomal dominant mutation in the fibrillin gene in chromosome 15. This can be inherited or sporadic. It causes arachnodactyly, high arched palate, wide arm-span, scoliosis and pes planus. Complications include upwards lens dislocation, aortic valve regurgitation, aortic dissection and pneumothorax.

An autosomal dominant mutation in the collagen gene can cause Ehlers-Danlos syndrome, which causes joint hypermobility leading to subluxation, hyperextension, sprains, dislocations and early onset osteoarthritis. The skin is fragile and bruises easily. Other complications include aortic valve regurgitation, aortic dissection and subarachnoid haemorrhage.

X-linked recessive mutation in the collagen type IV gene causes Alport's syndrome, which consists of bilateral sensorineural deafness, and chronic kidney disease that eventually requires a kidney transplant.

Overexpression of the IGF-2 gene causes Beckwith-Wiedemann syndrome. This presents at birth with macrosomia, organomegaly, macroglossia, microcephaly, hypoglycaemia and feeding difficulty.

Autosomal dominant mutation in the vHL tumour suppressor gene is responsible for causing von-Hippel Lindau syndrome. This is characterised by bilateral renal cell carcinomas, phaeochromocytoma, and both cerebellar and retinal haemangioblastomas.

27. A
Paracetamol

This lady has developed osteoarthritis in her knee. This is evident because of her pain, which worsens with use. On examination she has evidence of an effusion, joint swelling, stiffness, crepitus and a reduced range of movement. Conservative options for treatment include physiotherapy, weight loss and walking aids. If these are insufficient then analgesia should be started. All patients would begin at the bottom of the analgesic ladder with paracetamol, and only if this is insufficient should they be moved on to non-steroidal anti-inflammatory drugs (NSAIDs), weak opioids and finally strong opioids.

In liver cirrhosis paracetamol is the safest form of analgesia. NSAIDs should be avoided because they increase the risk of gastrointestinal bleeding. Also they can exacerbate renal disease, and these patients are already at risk of hepatorenal syndrome.

Opioids can precipitate hepatic encephalopathy by causing constipation, and codeine phosphate is one of the worst culprits for this. Opioids can also lead to sedation and confusion. Codeine is a pro-drug and needs to be metabolised by the liver to become active. Therefore its activity in liver disease is unpredictable.

Glucosamine sulfate is a dietary supplement that is marketed to support the structure and function of joints. However there is a lack of evidence to support this claim and therefore it is no longer recommended as treatment for osteoarthritis.

A total knee replacement is a last resort. It should only be used if all other treatments have failed.

28. D
Alendronic acid and lanzoprazole

Two important side effects of long-term corticosteroid use are peptic ulceration and osteoporosis. Therefore most patients who are due to start long-term steroids are prescribed a proton pump inhibitor (lanzoprazole) and a bisphosphonate (alendronic acid) as prophylaxis.

Other important side effects include hypertension, insulin resistance, abdominal obesity, proximal muscle wasting, cataracts, glaucoma, thinning of the skin and immunosuppression.

Alfacalcidiol is an active vitamin D supplement. It can be combined with calcium supplements to treat osteomalacia and osteopenia (which is a less severe version of osteoporosis).

Captorpil is an angiotensin converting enzyme (ACE) inhibitor used to treat hypertension and metformin is a biguanide used to treat type 2 diabetes mellitus. Although both hypertension and diabetes mellitus can result from long-term corticosteroid use, these drugs are not given as prophylaxis.

Raloxifene is a selective oestrogen receptor modulator used to treat osteoporosis. It is used as a second line treatment if a bisphosphonate can't be tolerated. Ranitidine is an H_2-receptor antagonist used to reduce gastric acid secretion.

Magnesium trisilicate is an antacid, and gliclazide is a sulphonylurea. Neither of these drugs would be used as prophylaxis in this scenario.

29. E
Psoriatic arthritis

Psoriatic arthritis is one of the seronegative spondyloarthritides and is associated with the development of a psoriatic rash. The joint pathology can present before the rash, and have a variety of different patterns of presentation. It can be a symmetrical polyarthritis, just affect the distal interphalangeal joints, an asymmetrical oligoarthritis, spinal involvement or psoriatic arthritis mutilans (which is a severe deformity caused by destruction and shortening of the phalageal bones). Erosive changes in psoriatic arthritis cause a classic 'pencil in cup' X-ray appearance.

Rheumatoid arthritis classically spares the distal interphalangeal joints; therefore this is less likely to be the underlying diagnosis.

Systemic lupus erythematosus (SLE) doesn't normally cause radiological changes, because it causes a non-erosive arthropathy.

Enteropathic arthropathy is also one of the seronegative spondyloarthritides, but would present with gastrointestinal symptoms as well as joint pain.

30. B
Loss of sensation on the dorsal lateral aspect of the foot

This patient has developed sciatica. This is where a prolapsed vertebral disc causes compression of the sciatic nerve roots. This results in back pain that radiates down the leg and can be reproduced by a straight leg raise. The most common sites for a prolapsed disc are between L4 and L5, or between S1 and S2. This patient has developed an L4-L5 prolapse, which has affected the sensation in the L5 dermatome, which is on the lateral dorsal aspect of the foot.

Perianal anaesthesia occurs in cauda equina syndrome. This presents with back pain, asymmetrical leg pain, loss of reflexes, atrophy and flaccid paralysis. There is also reduced anal sphincter tone.

Upward going planters would occur as a result of an upper motor neurone lesion, which could be present in the brain or the spine. Spinal cord compression would cause back pain and upper motor neurone signs below the level of the lesion including weakness, hypertonia and hyperreflexia.

Urinary retention could occur in both spinal cord compression and conus medullaris lesions. Conus medullaris lesions cause a mix of upper and lower motor neurone signs, urinary retention and constipation.

Erosive changes on a lumbar spine X-ray may be seen in severe joint conditions. The radiological changes take a while to develop, and wouldn't be present in the first acute flare.

Surgery Questions

1. A 60-year-old presents with abdominal pain, which radiates to her back. This has been ongoing for a week. Her past medical history includes atrial fibrillation for which she takes warfarin. On examination there is diffuse abdominal tenderness, but there is no guarding or rebound tenderness, and the rectal exam is unremarkable with no melaena present. Her observations are stable. Initial blood tests reveal that she is anaemic and her international normalised ratio (INR) is above the therapeutic range. What is the most likely underlying diagnosis?

A. Ruptured abdominal aortic aneurysm
B. Renal stone
C. Perforated duodenal ulcer
D. Retroperitoneal haematoma
E. Pancreatitis

2. A 22-year-old male presents to hospital with abdominal pain, which started in the umbilical region but is now localised to the right iliac fossa. He has anorexia and a fever. There is localised guarding and on palpation a tender mass can be felt in the right iliac fossa. Which of the following is most likely to be used in the initial management of this patient?

A. Urgent appendicectomy
B. Intravenous cefuroxime and metronidazole
C. Gastroenterology referral
D. Ultrasound guided drain
E. Discharge and follow-up with his general practitioner (GP)

3. A 75-year-old patient with known atrial fibrillation presents to hospital with severe diffuse abdominal pain and tenderness. The patient is hypotensive and tachycardic. Initial blood tests show an increasing serum lactate and a raised serum amylase. Which of the following investigations is most useful in confirming the underlying diagnosis?

A. Ultrasound scan of the abdomen
B. Computed tomography (CT) angiography of the abdomen and pelvis
C. Electrocardiogram (ECG), abdominal X-ray and erect chest X-ray
D. Colonoscopy with biopsy
E. Faecal serology

4. A 65-year-old alcoholic male presents to his doctor with a dull epigastric pain. On further questioning he reveals recent weight loss and worsening diarrhoea, which he describes as pale and difficult to flush. He describes his urine as being dark and he recently developed a widespread itch. Which of the following investigations is most accurate in confirming the underlying diagnosis?

A. Endoscopic sonography
B. Ultrasound scan of the abdomen
C. Serum amylase
D. Serum CA19-9
E. Liver function tests (LFTs) with gamma-glutamyl transferase (GGT)

5. Which of the following is the greatest risk factor for developing colorectal cancer?

A. Age
B. Smoking
C. Ulcerative colitis
D. Hereditary non-polyposis colorectal cancer (HNPCC)
E. Familial adenomatous polyposis

6. An elderly lady presents to her doctor with tiredness and weight loss. Initial blood tests show she has a mild microcytic anaemia and as a result is sent for an urgent colonoscopy. This reveals a mass present in the upper part of the sigmoid colon. Which of the following should occur next in this patient's management?

A. Sigmoid colectomy
B. Pre-operative radiotherapy
C. Serum alpha-fetoprotein
D. Computed tomography (CT) scan of the chest, abdomen and pelvis
E. Admission to hospital for a blood transfusion

7. A patient is diagnosed with colorectal cancer. The mass is found to have invaded through the full thickness of the muscularis propria without involving any lymph nodes. What Dukes stage is this cancer?

A. Dukes A
B. Dukes B1
C. Dukes B2
D. Dukes C1
E. Dukes C2

8. A 50-year-old woman presents with colicky right upper quadrant pain, which radiates to her shoulder. It is associated with nausea and vomiting. On examination her observations are normal and there is yellowing of her sclera. Which of the following is the most likely diagnosis?

A. Biliary colic
B. Acute cholecystitis
C. Choledocholithiasis
D. Ascending cholangitis
E. Gallbladder empyema

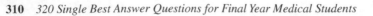
9. A 50-year-old overweight female patient was recently started on hormone replacement therapy as she is going through the menopause. She presented to her hospital with colicky right upper quadrant pain, which radiated to her shoulder. She also described having a fever and rigors for the past few days. On monitoring her temperature the nurses noted various spikes. On examination there was abdominal tenderness but no jaundice. Which of the following is the most likely diagnosis?

A. Acute drug induced hepatitis
B. Liver abscess
C. Gallbladder mucocoele
D. Gallbladder empyema
E. Ascending cholangitis

10. A 70-year-old man returns to the ward following a trans-urethral resection of the prostate (TURP). He rapidly loses consciousness and starts having uncontrolled rhythmic tonic clonic movements of his arms and legs. Which of the following is most likely to be the cause of his symptoms?

A. Withdrawal of anaesthetic drugs
B. Hyponatraemia
C. Hypernatraemia
D. Hypocalcaemia
E. Uraemia

11. Following surgery on her oesophagus a patient was returned to the ward for monitoring. She initially vomited and this was followed by severe retching and severe abdominal pain. The junior doctor was unable to pass an nasogastric (NG) tube, despite three attempts. What is the most likely underlying diagnosis?

A. Oesophageal adhesion
B. Boerhaave syndrome
C. Zenker's diverticulum
D. Gastric volvulus
E. Achalasia

12. A 24-year-old man has just undergone a terminal ileal resection as part of treatment for Crohn's disease. Which of the following could occur as a result of this operation?

A   Microcytic anaemia
B. Folate deficiency
C. Beriberi
D. Renal stones
E. Scurvy

13. Which of the following nerves is most at risk of being damaged following a shoulder dislocation?

A. Axillary nerve
B. Median nerve
C. Ulnar nerve
D. Radial nerve
E. Accessory nerve

14. A 55-year-old lady is diagnosed with breast cancer and subsequently has the tumour removed with breast conserving surgery. A couple of weeks later she notices a painless lump beneath the incision. On examination she is apyrexial, the lump is non-tender, firm and well circumscribed. Initial blood tests show her serum CA 15-3 is undetectable. What is the most likely diagnosis?

A. Recurrence of the breast cancer
B. Abscess
C. Fibroadenoma
D. Fat necrosis
E. Cystic disease

15. A 50-year-old smoker presents to her general practitioner (GP) with nipple discharge. On examination there is green discharge from the nipple and no lumps were palpable. Which of the following investigations is most likely to be used to confirm the underlying diagnosis?

A. Serum CA 15-3
B. Ultrasound scan
C. Breast mammogram
D. Computed tomography (CT) scan of the chest
E. Ultrasound guided core biopsy

16. A 22-year-old lady presents to hospital with right iliac fossa pain. On examination there is localised guarding and rebound tenderness. Which of the following sets of investigations should be carried out first?

A. Urinary beta-human chorionic gonadotropin (hCG)
B. Erect chest X-ray
C. Computed tomography (CT) scan of the abdomen
D. Full blood count and serum c-reactive protein (CRP)
E. Liver function tests (LFTs) with gamma-glutamyl transferase (GGT)

17. A 45-year-old lady presents to her doctor with a unilateral erythematous, itchy rash around her nipple. She has already tried using emollients, but these haven't helped. On examination her nipple is inverted. Which of the following is the most likely diagnosis?

A. Nipple eczema
B. Ductal carcinoma in-situ
C. Lobular carcinoma in-situ
D. Medullary carcinoma
E. Infective mastitis

18. A patient who has a history of Crohn's disease and resection of the terminal ileum presents with abdominal pain and distention. He is has been constipated for 4 days and began vomiting today. Which of the following is the most important next step in this patient's management?

A. Prescription of an antiemetic
B. Insertion of a nasogastric tube and intravenous fluids
C. Rigid sigmoidoscopy and air insufflation
D. Intravenous cefuroxime and metronidazole
E. Intravenous neostigmine

19. A 70-year-old male presents with severe abdominal pain, distention, absolute constipation and vomiting. You are asked to prescribe him an antiemetic. Which of the following drugs is contraindicated in this patient?

A. Dexamethasone
B. Cyclizine
C. Ondansetron
D. Hyoscine butylbromide
E. Metoclopramide

20. A 70-year-old patient returns to the ward after a right hemicolectomy. Five days later he complains of cramping abdominal pains, and he has been unable to open his bowels since the surgery. Which of the following is the most likely underlying cause of his symptoms?

A. Adhesions
B. Paralytic ileus
C. Pseudo-obstruction
D. Caecal volvulus
E. Recurrence of colorectal cancer

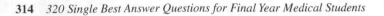

21. An 18-year-old patient has a smooth lump on the left side of his neck. It is situated in the anterior triangle, under the anterior border of the sternocleidomastoid muscle and roughly one third of the way down the sternocleidomastoid muscle. Which of the following is the most likely diagnosis?

A. Thyroglossal cyst
B. Branchial cleft cyst
C. Carotid artery aneurysm
D. Dermoid cyst
E. Chondroma

22. Following parotid surgery to remove a pleomorphic adenoma a patient presents complaining of facial flushing. She states that whenever she is eating she develops an erythematous rash on her cheek and starts sweating. She also experiences a burning pain in the distribution of the rash. What is the most likely underlying diagnosis?

A. Facial nerve palsy
B. Salivary fistula
C. Staphylococcal infection
D. Heerfordt's syndrome
E. Frey's syndrome

23. A patient is scheduled to have a routine operation. He is due to have his general anaesthetic at 2 pm. When is the latest time he should be told to stop eating food?

A. 6 am
B. 7 am
C. 8 am
D. 9 am
E. 10 am

24. A patient with type 1 diabetes is admitted for routine surgical operation, which is due to take 2 hours and requires general anaesthesia. He currently takes actrapid before meals three times a day and lantus before going to sleep. Which of the following regimes should be used to manage his blood glucose levels once he starts fasting?

A. Stop all subcutaneous insulin and start an intravenous insulin sliding scale

B. Stop all subcutaneous insulin and start a fixed rate intravenous insulin infusion

C. Start an intravenous 5% dextrose infusion and give the normal subcutaneous insulin regime

D. Give the normal subcutaneous insulin regime along with an intravenous insulin sliding scale

E. Stop the subcutaneous actrapid, continue to give subcutaneous lantus, and start an intravenous insulin sliding scale

25. A 65-year-old male presents to his doctor with a dull back ache that has been worsening over the last 3 months. On examination a pulsatile and expansile mass can be felt at the level of the umbilicus. Which of the following investigations would be most sensitive in confirming the underlying diagnosis?

A. Abdominal X-ray

B. Abdominal ultrasound

C. Computed tomography (CT) scan of the abdomen

D. Ankle brachial pressure index

E. Computed tomography (CT) venogram

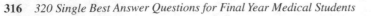

26. A 60-year-old man with a history of ischaemic heart disease presents to his doctor with pain in his legs. He states that he gets cramping pains in his buttocks and thighs when he tries to exercise. On systems review he reluctantly reveals he has also developed erectile dysfunction. On examination his femoral pulses are absent and there is wasting of his thighs and buttocks. Which of the following conditions has caused this patient's symptoms?

A. Aortoiliac occlusive disease
B. Peripheral artery disease affecting both femoral arteries
C. Cauda equina syndrome
D. Inferior vena cava thrombosis
E. Abdominal aortic aneurysm

27. A 60-year-old male is diagnosed with an abdominal aortic aneurysm following an asymptomatic screen. It is 4 cm in diameter. Which of the following is the best form of management for this patient?

A. No further treatment required
B. Annual ultrasound scans of the abdomen
C. Annual computed tomography (CT) scans of the abdomen
D. Open surgical repair
E. Endovascular aneurysm repair (EVAR)

28. A patient presents to his doctor with a burning sensation in this thigh. It is confined to the anterolateral area of his left thigh and is accompanied by periods of numbness and paraesthesia. On examination he has normal strength throughout both legs. Which of the following is the most likely underlying diagnosis?

A. Diabetic amyotrophy
B. Complex regional pain syndrome type 1
C. Complex regional pain syndrome type 2
D. Femoral nerve compression
E. Meralgia paraesthetica

9"x6"
b3668_04-Haematology.indd 129
b3668   320 Single Best Answer Questions for Final Year Medical Students
23-Aug-19 6:

29. An 18-year-old man presents with knee pain. This came on suddenly as a sharp pain while he was turning quickly during a football match one week ago. Since then his knee has been swollen, he has been unable to completely straighten his leg, and has experienced painful locking of his knee. Which of the following is the most likely diagnosis?

A. Osteoarthritis
B. Anterior cruciate ligament tear
C. Meniscal tear
D. Patella tendon rupture
E. Suprapatella effusion

30. A 16-year-old male presents with ongoing pain around his knee. On examination there is clear localised swelling and tenderness. An X-ray of the knee shows periosteal elevation (known as Codman's triangle) and underlying bone destruction with new bone formation, described as 'sunray spicules'. Which of the following is the most likely underlying condition?

A. Ewing's sarcoma
B. Osteosarcoma
C. Giant cell tumour
D. Secondary metastases to the bone cortex
E. Osgood-Schlatter disease

31. Which of the following is the greatest risk factor for breast cancer?

A. Previous use of a mirena coil
B. Multiple pregnancies
C. Going through the menopause at 45 years old
D. Menarche at 10 years old
E. A body mass index of 27

Surgery Answers

1. D
Retroperitoneal haematoma

This is an accumulation of blood in the retroperitoneal space. It can be caused by anticoagulation, a ruptured abdominal aortic aneurysm, a ruptured renal aneurysm and malignancy. The clinical features may vary depending on how much blood has accumulated. Classically it would present with abdominal or flank pain and anaemia.

All the conditions listed above cause abdominal pain that can radiate to the back. The reason being, that they all involve retroperitoneal structures.

A ruptured abdominal aortic aneurysm would present with sudden onset pain, hypotension and tachycardia. This would cause the patient to become unstable very quickly.

A renal stone would present with a colicky pain in the flank that radiates to the groin and may be accompanied by urinary symptoms and haematuria. However it wouldn't cause anaemia.

A perforated duodenal ulcer would lead to an upper gastrointestinal bleed, causing haematemesis and melaena. The blood loss would cause anaemia and if severe would lead to hypovolaemic shock.

Pancreatitis would present with epigastric pain, diarrhoea, nausea and vomiting. Signs would include Grey Turner's sign (which is bruising of the flanks) and Cullen's sign (which is bruising around the umbilicus).

9"x6"
b3668_04-Haematology.indd   131
b3668   320 Single Best Answer Questions for Final Year Medical Students
23-Aug-19 6:

Surgery Answers   319

2. B
Intravenous cefuroxime and metronidazole

This patient has developed an appendix mass, which is where the appendix becomes inflamed and adheres to the overlying omentum and small bowel. It presents in a similar manner to appendicitis, but often presents over a longer duration. Patients with an appendix mass are treated with antibiotics to begin with. The reason being that at this point the inflammation surrounding the appendix would make an appendicectomy too difficult to perform. Patients are brought back into hospital once the inflammation has settled for an elective appendicectomy.

If this patient just had an uncomplicated appendicitis, without a palpable mass then an urgent appendicectomy would be the correct answer.

Patients with an appendix mass require intravenous antibiotics to begin with and therefore immediate discharge wouldn't be recommended.

Despite it being treated medically an appendix mass is something that can be dealt with on a surgical ward and doesn't require referral to gastroenterology.

A further complication of appendicitis is an appendix abscess. Patients often are investigated by use of a computed tomography (CT) scan, and at this point any abscess formation would be identified. If this were the case then ultrasound-guided drainage would be appropriate. However antibiotics would still be started first. Classically an abscess would cause a swinging fever with various spikes in temperature.

3. B
Computed tomography (CT) angiography of the abdomen and pelvis

This patient has developed mesenteric ischaemia. This should be suspected in any patient who has atrial fibrillation and presents with abdominal pain, as atrial fibrillation can cause systemic emboli. It presents with severe abdominal pain, hypovolaemic shock and a lack of abdominal signs. These patients are often very sick, but with few clinical signs. Blood tests may show raised haemoglobin due to plasma loss, raised white cell count, moderately raised serum amylase and a rising serum lactate, along with a metabolic acidosis. The diagnosis can be confirmed by arteriography or CT angiography, but most are made during a laparotomy, which reveals areas of necrotic bowel.

Other causes of mesenteric ischaemia include arterial thrombosis, venous thrombosis, trauma, vasculitis and strangulation.

An ultrasound scan of the abdomen could be used to identify large masses, evidence of ureteric obstruction and assess the integrity of the liver, but would not be able to identify mesenteric ischaemia.

An ECG would confirm the presence of atrial fibrillation. In mesenteric ischaemia an abdominal X-ray would show a 'gassless' abdomen and may show 'thumb-printing' as a result of inflammation and oedema. However, it wouldn't confirm the underlying cause. An erect chest X-ray would be useful to look for any signs of perforation, but wouldn't confirm the underlying cause.

Colonoscopy and biopsy would be used to diagnose colorectal cancer.

Faecal serology would be used if an infective cause were suspected.

4. A
Endoscopic sonography

This patient has presented with signs and symptoms consistent with obstructive jaundice. He describes having dark urine, pale stools and puritis. In a patient with a history of alcohol misuse the most likely diagnosis in this case is pancreatic cancer. Further aspects of the history that make this more likely are the dull epigastric pain, steatorrhea (stool that is difficult to flush) and the recent weight loss. Endoscopic sonography would show a mass at the head of the pancreas, along with a dilated biliary tree, and is the most accurate diagnostic investigation.

An ultrasound scan of the abdomen is unlikely to visualise the pancreas well and therefore would not be a reliable investigation in diagnosing pancreatic cancer.

Serum amylase is a non-specific blood test, which can be raised in a number of conditions such as acute pancreatitis, mesenteric ischaemia, perforated peptic ulcer, diabetic ketoacidosis, chronic kidney disease and mumps. It is useful in acute pancreatitis because it is often extremely raised, but it wouldn't be used to confirm a diagnosis of pancreatic cancer.

Serum CA19-9 is a tumour marker for pancreatic cancer. Like all tumour markers, it is not very specific and therefore can't be used to confirm an underlying diagnosis.

Liver function tests (LFTs) with gamma-glutamyl transferase (GGT) would be useful, and would show a cholestatic picture (raised alkaline phosphatase [ALP], raised GGT and raised conjugated bilirubin). It would confirm the presence of obstructive jaundice, but wouldn't confirm the underlying cause.

5. E
Familial adenomatous polyposis

Familial adenomatous polyposis is an autosomal dominant condition caused by a mutation in the APC gene, which leads to numerous adenomatous polyps forming in the colon. These start as benign polyps but eventually become malignant. Almost all of these patients will develop colon cancer by the age of 50. In many cases this condition is treated with a prophylactic total colectomy before colorectal cancer develops. All the other conditions listed are also risk factors for developing colorectal cancer.

6. D
Computed tomography (CT) scan of the chest, abdomen and pelvis

This patient has colorectal cancer. The next step in her management is to stage the cancer, therefore a CT scan of the chest, abdomen and pelvis is required to look for any metastases. Once the cancer has been staged the next step in treatment may be decided. This could involve pre-operative radiotherapy, which may be used in rectal cancer to reduce the size of the tumour. In rectal cancer it has also been shown to increase rates of survival. If there are no distant metastases, a sigmoid colectomy is the mainstay of treatment in sigmoid cancer.

Serum alpha-fetoprotein is a tumour marker, which can be raised in hepatocellular carcinoma; therefore it is not useful in the diagnosis or treatment of colorectal cancer. The tumour marker used in colorectal cancer is carcinoembryonic antigen (CEA).

This patient would only require a blood transfusion if she had severe or symptomatic anaemia. Therefore at this point it is unlikely to be required.

7. C
Dukes B2

Dukes staging is specific to colorectal cancer.

Dukes A: Cancer is limited to the mucosa

Dukes B1: Cancer has extended into the muscularis propria, but not extended through it, and no lymph nodes are involved.

Dukes B2: Cancer has extended through the muscularis propria, and no lymph nodes are involved.

Dukes C1: Cancer has extended into the muscularis propria, but not extended through it and lymph nodes are involved.

Dukes C2: Cancer has extended through the muscularis propria, and lymph nodes are involved.

Dukes D: There is distant metastatic spread.

8. C
Choledocholithiasis

Choledocholithiasis is the presence of a gallstone in the common bile duct. It presents with biliary colic and obstructive jaundice. It can eventually result in ascending cholangitis, which presents with Charcot's triad (jaundice, fever and right upper quadrant pain), and can cause acute pancreatitis. This case is unlikely to have progressed to ascending cholangitis yet, because this patient has stable observations and is apyrexial.

Biliary colic presents with colicky right upper quadrant pain, which worsens on eating fatty foods. It doesn't cause a fever or jaundice.

Acute cholecystitis also presents with colicky right upper quadrant pain, nausea and vomiting, and it can also cause a fever. On examination Murphy's sign may be present. It doesn't cause jaundice.

A gallbladder empyema can occur as a complication of a gallstone, and would present with colicky right upper quadrant pain and a spiking temperature.

9. D
Gallbladder empyema

A gallbladder empyema is a complication that can occur as a result of a gallstone. The gallstone can lead to blockage of the gallbladder neck, and result in a build up of fluid within the gallbladder. If this becomes infected it causes an empyema which presents with right upper quadrant pain and a spiking temperature. Hormone replacement therapy is a risk factor for developing cholesterol gallstones. Other risk factors include female gender, age, obesity, the combined oral contraceptive pill and fibrates. Haemolysis can lead to formation of pigment gallstones.

A gallbladder mucocoele is a build up of mucus within the gallbladder and is another complication of a gallstone. It can precede formation of an empyema, but wouldn't cause a fever or rigors.

Ascending cholangitis would present with Charcot's triad (jaundice, fever and right upper quadrant pain). This patient is not jaundiced making this diagnosis unlikely.

Acute drug induced hepatitis may cause right upper quadrant pain, but this is likely to be a constant pain, rather than colicky. Causes would include paracetamol overdose, rifampicin, isoniazid, pyrazinamide, statins, sodium valproate and halothane.

A liver abscess would present with right upper quadrant pain, hepatomegaly and a spiking temperature. This may occur following travel to a foreign country and is far less common than gallstone pathology.

10. B
Hyponatraemia

This patient has developed post-TURP syndrome. This is caused by systemic absorption of the irrigation fluids used during the procedure and these lead to dilution of the plasma, hyponatraemia and hypothermia. The presence of hyponatraemia can lead to seizures. The manifestations of post-TURP syndrome ranges from mild (restlessness, nausea, shortness of breath, and dizziness) to severe (seizures, coma, bradycardia, and cardiovascular collapse).

11. D
Gastric volvulus

This patient has developed a gastric volvulus, which is where the stomach becomes twisted on its axis and leads to gastro-oesophageal obstruction. It can occur as a result of congenital conditions (paraoseophageal hernias, congenital bands, pyloric stenosis) or following gastric/oesophageal surgery. It presents with pain and vomiting followed by retching and failed attempts to pass a nasogastric tube.

Oesophageal adhesions are extremely uncommon, and would occur a few months after surgery.

Boerhaave syndrome is oesophageal rupture secondary to violent emesis. It would present with odynophagea, surgical emphysema, tachypnoea and shock.

Zenker's diverticulum is also known as a pharyngeal pouch. This would present with dysphagia, halitosis, a fluctuant mass in the neck, which becomes enlarged when eating and auscultation of the mass often reveals a gurgling sound.

Achalasia is where the lower oesophageal sphincter fails to relax resulting in dysphagia and regurgitation.

12. D
Renal stones

The terminal ileum is the only area of the digestive system that can absorb bile salts and vitamin B12. Therefore terminal ileal resection would cause vitamin B12 deficiency (not folate deficiency as this can be absorbed elsewhere) and a macrocytic megaloblastic anaemia (not microcytic). The lack of bile salt reabsorption means that lipids cannot be absorbed. The excess lipids in the small intestine bind to calcium ions, thus preventing the calcium ions from binding to oxalate. Therefore there is increased absorption of oxalate, which results in renal stones.

Scurvy occurs as a result of vitamin C deficiency and presents with gingivitis, bleeding from the gums, nose and hair follicles, muscle pains and weakness, and oedema.

Beriberi occurs as a result of thiamine deficiency and can be either 'wet beriberi', which causes a high output cardiac failure or 'dry beriberi' which causes a neuropathy.

13. E
Axillary nerve

The axillary nerve passes around the neck of the humerus, so any displacement of the proximal humerus can lead to damage to the axillary nerve. In any patient who has dislocated their shoulder it is important to check sensation over the C5 dermatome.

14. D
Fat necrosis

Fat necrosis is where trauma has led to fibrosis and calcification of the breast tissue. It can occur following surgery. It may be difficult to differentiate clinically from breast cancer. This is the most likely diagnosis in this patient as she has just recently had breast surgery. Recurrence of breast cancer is unlikely to occur that quickly after surgery. Also her tumour marker is undetectable. Tumour markers cannot be used to make a diagnosis; but they are a good test for monitoring recurrence.

An abscess could occur following surgery, but would present with a painful lump, and the patient would be febrile.

Fibroadenomas are benign masses formed from the overgrowth of the mesenchymal tissue in the breast. They are firm, smooth and mobile. They grow slowly and are more common in younger adults.

Breast cysts are a common cause of breast lumps and are fluid filled sacs that are benign in nature. They are often fluctuant and change in characteristics depending on the stage of the menstrual cycle.

15. C
Breast mammogram

This patient has developed duct ectasia, which is a breast condition caused by the ducts becoming blocked due to stasis of colostrum. It can present with nipple inversion, pain and green/bloody discharge. Smoking is the main risk factor for duct ectasia, and it becomes more common with age. Diagnosis is made by use of a mammogram, which would show dilated breast ducts.

CA 15-3 is a tumour marker for breast cancer, and would be used to monitor breast cancer treatment, but not to make a diagnosis. If a diagnosis of breast cancer was suspected it would be confirmed by use of an ultrasound guided biopsy or fine needle aspiration. However this diagnosis would be less likely in this patient as no lump is palpable.

An ultrasound scan is used to investigate breast pathology in younger patients, because their breasts are far denser, and a mammogram would be unable to visualise the pathology accurately.

A CT scan of the chest would be used as part of a staging process if a diagnosis of breast cancer were made, along with a CT scan of the abdomen and pelvis.

16. A
Urinary beta-human chorionic gonadotropin (hCG)

Any female patient who is presenting with abdominal pain should have a pregnancy test carried out. This patient has presented with classic signs of appendicitis, however before further investigations are to be carried out the possibility of an ectopic pregnancy should be ruled out first.

An erect chest X-ray would be used to rule out perforation by looking for air under the diaphragm.

To confirm a diagnosis of appendicitis, a CT scan of the abdomen is often requested before carrying out an operation.

FBC and CRP would both be used to look for evidence of inflammation and infection.

17. B
Ductal carcinoma in-situ

This patient has developed Paget's disease of the breast, which is caused by an underlying ductal carcinoma in-situ. It presents with a unilateral erythematous rash around the nipple, which doesn't respond to normal eczema treatment (such as emollients). There may also be nipple retraction and inversion, and straw-coloured discharge.

Lobular carcinoma in-situ doesn't present with a rash around the nipple. The main differences are that it tends to be multifocal and there is no micro-calcification seen on the mammogram. Also lobular carcinoma in-situ mainly occurs in pre-menopausal women, whereas ductal carcinoma in-situ occurs in both pre and post-menopausal women.

A medullary carcinoma is a rare form of breast cancer, which mainly tends to affect younger women.

Infective mastitis commonly occurs in women who are breast-feeding. It can present with a painful, red swollen area of breast tissue, a fever and nipple discharge.

Nipple eczema is often bilateral, and would respond to treatment with emollients. If it is severe topical corticosteroids may be required.

18. B
Insertion of a nasogastric tube and intravenous fluids

This patient has developed bowel obstruction, which is likely to have occurred from adhesions that have resulted from his previous surgery. Once a diagnosis of obstruction is made a patient should immediately be made 'nil by mouth'. A nasogastric tube should be inserted to aspirate gastric fluid, decompress the bowel and allow the bowel to rest and intravenous fluids are also essential.

An antiemetic may be prescribed, but the best way to prevent vomiting is to insert a nasogastric tube and aspirate the gastric contents. Therefore an antiemetic is not essential.

Rigid sigmoidoscopy and air insufflation is used to treat a sigmoid volvulus. Firstly it is more likely this patient has small bowel obstruction as a result of adhesions, due to their history. Secondly even if a volvulus were the cause of obstruction in this patient, the immediate management would still be insertion of a nasogastric tube and intravenous fluids.

Intravenous cefuroxime and metronidazole is a common combination of antibiotics used during abdominal surgery, both as prophylaxis and to treat infections that may complicate surgery. However it is not required in this case.

Neostigmine is an acetylcholinesterase inhibitor, which can be used to increase gut motility in a paralytic ileus. However even in a paralytic ileus the first measure would be to insert a nasogastric tube and give intravenous fluids.

19. E
Metoclopramide

This patient has developed bowel obstruction. This classically presents with abdominal distention, colicky pain, absolute constipation and vomiting. Metoclopramide and domperidone are both dopamine D2-receptor antagonists, and have pro-kinetic properties. They are contraindicated in obstruction because they can increase the risk of perforation. The other antiemetics are all safe in bowel obstruction.

20. B
Paralytic ileus

A paralytic ileus is an adynamic bowel that occurs due to a lack of normal peristaltic contractions within the intestines. It presents with obstruction and absent bowel sounds. Common causes include abdominal surgery, spinal surgery, any cause of localised peritonitis such as pancreatitis, electrolyte imbalances (hypokalaemia, hyponatraemia, uraemia) and drugs (opiates, antimuscarinics, tricyclic antidepressants).

Pseudo-obstruction is like a mechanical obstruction where no cause is found.

Adhesions are a common cause of obstruction, but would occur months (not days) after surgery.

Caecal volvulus is a cause of colonic obstruction, but wouldn't occur after a right hemicolectomy, as the caecum would have been removed.

Recurrence of colorectal cancer is always a possibility if the tumour was not correctly resected, but this would take months to manifest.

21. B
Branchial cleft cyst

A branchial cleft cyst is a congenital cyst that arises due to either failure to obliterate the second branchial cleft, or due to failure of the fusion of the second and third branchial clefts. It presents with a fluctuant lump on the side of the neck, at the level where the upper third of the sternocleido-mastoid muscle meets the middle third of sternocleidomastoid muscle.

A thyroglossal cyst is a cyst that forms from a persistent remnant of the thyroglossal duct. It presents as a midline neck lump, which moves upwards when the patient protrudes their tongue.

Carotid artery aneurysms are pulsatile expansile masses that are found in the anterior triangle of the neck.

A dermoid cyst is a midline lump which often occurs in young patients, and when excised contains dermal structures, such as teeth or hair.

A chondroma is a benign cartilaginous tumour, which can form a hard lump in the midline of the neck.

22. E
Frey's syndrome

Frey's syndrome is a condition that occurs following trauma to the parotid gland. Normally the auriculo-temporal branch of the trigeminal nerve sends parasympathetic fibres to the parotid gland, and sympathetic fibres to the facial sweat glands. Trauma to this area means that these nerves must then re-grow, and often they switch places. This results in gustatory sweating, meaning that when the patient eats the sweat glands on the cheek become stimulated, resulting in sweating and erythema.

Facial nerve palsy can occur following trauma to the parotid gland as the facial nerve passes through the gland on its way to supply the facial muscles. However this would cause a unilateral facial droop and facial muscle weakness. There may also be a loss of taste in the anterior two thirds of the tongue and hyperacusis due to stapedius muscle paralysis.

Salivary fistulas can occur following parotid surgery and its presentation will depend on where the fistula communicates. If it communicates with the mouth there are often no symptoms, but if it communicates with the skin it can cause leakage of saliva onto the skin, which may impair healing after surgery.

A Staphylococcal infection of the parotid gland can occur as a result of surgery or due to an infection tracking up from an infected tooth. It presents with painful swelling and a fever.

Heerfordt's syndrome is a rare manifestation of sarcoidosis, which consists of acute sarcoidosis, with uveitis and salivary or lacrimal gland swelling.

23. C
8 am

For all adult elective surgery requiring general anaesthesia, healthy patients who don't have any known gastrointestinal pathology are required to stop eating food 6 hours before their procedure and stop drinking fluids 2 hours before.

24. E
Stop the subcutaneous actrapid, continue to give subcutaneous lantus and start an intravenous insulin sliding scale

The best management of type 1 diabetes once a patient becomes 'nil by mouth' is to use an insulin sliding scale. It has also been shown that to prevent large spikes in the patient's insulin requirements their basal long acting insulin should be continued. This also makes it easier to restart the patient's insulin regime once they are able to resume normal eating habits.

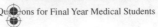
25. C
Computed tomography (CT) scan of the abdomen

This patent has an abdominal aortic aneurysm. The most sensitive scan used to make a diagnosis is a CT scan of the abdomen.

An abdominal ultrasound is now used for screening, however even if this test is positive, patients are still sent for a CT scan of the abdomen to confirm the diagnosis.

An abdominal X-ray would often be normal; however sometimes if an aneurysm is chronic, there may be evidence of calcification around the walls of the aneurysm.

Ankle brachial pressure index (ABPI) is used to diagnose peripheral vascular disease.

CT venogram is a scan used to identify thrombosis in the veins.

26. A
Aortoiliac occlusive disease

This patient has developed Leriche syndrome, which is caused by peripheral artery disease affecting the abdominal aorta or the common iliac arteries. It presents with a triad of features: claudication in the buttocks and thighs, absent or decreased femoral pulses and erectile dysfunction.

Peripheral artery disease affecting both femoral arteries would cause claudication in the thighs, but not the buttocks. Also depending on the level of occlusion the femoral arteries may still be palpable, but it is likely that the distal pulses will not be palpable unless collaterals have formed.

Cauda equina syndrome is caused by compression of the cauda equina (which is the lumbar and sacral plexus). This presents with back pain, asymmetrical leg pain and weakness, saddle anaesthesia, loss of sphincter tone and incontinence.

Inferior vena cava thrombosis causes venous hypertension, which leads to bilateral leg oedema, varicose veins and non-healing venous ulcers. Depending on its location it can also cause hepatomegaly and portal hypertension resulting in ascites, caput medusae, splenomegaly and varices. However many patents may only present when the thrombus has resulted in a pulmonary embolism.

Abdominal aortic aneurysms are often asymptomatic until they rupture, causing hypovolaemic shock. However sometimes they can cause back pain and compression of nearby abdominal organs.

27. B
Annual abdominal ultrasound scans

A screening program has now begun in the United Kingdom; so all males at the age of 65 years will have an abdominal ultrasound. If this shows evidence of an abdominal aortic aneurysm then it will be confirmed by use of a CT scan of the abdomen. The diameter of the aneurysm will determine the treatment pathway. If it is between 3 cm–4.4 cm then they will have an annual ultrasound. If it is between 4.5 cm–5.4 cm they will have a three monthly ultrasound scans and if it is 5.5 cm or larger then patients are considered for surgery. This can be open surgery or endovascular aneurysm repair (EVAR). EVAR has a reduced mortality in the first four years after surgery, but the longer-term outcomes are still unknown.

28. E
Meralgia paraesthetica

Meralgia paraesthetica is a condition caused by injury or compression of the lateral cutaneous nerve of the thigh as it passes beneath the inguinal ligament. It presents with pain on the lateral side of the thigh, which is often described as a burning or tingling sensation. This is often a self-limiting condition. However if medical management fails it may require surgical decompression.

Femoral nerve compression would result in weakness and wasting of the quadriceps muscles.

Diabetic amyotrophy is a painful wasting of the quadriceps and other pelvifemoral muscles, and is due to a neuropathy that can occur in uncontrolled diabetes mellitus.

Complex regional pain syndrome type 1 is a sequel to limb trauma without any evidence of nerve damage. Whereas complex regional pain syndrome type 2 occurs following limb injury and does have evidence of nerve injury. It typically presents with a burning pain, hyperalgesia, abnormal sweating and abnormal temperature control of the affected area. The overlying skin is often oedematous, shiny and atrophic.

29. C
Meniscal tear

A meniscal tear is a common sporting injury, which classically occurs during performing a sharp turn. It presents with pain and swelling of the knee. Patients complain of locking of the knee joint and a reduced range of movement. On examination an effusion may be present and McMurray's test may be positive. Performing a twisting motion during a McMurray's test often exacerbates the pain experienced by the patient, because it causes the meniscal fragment to get pinched.

An anterior cruciate ligament tear is also a common sporting injury. When the injury occurs patients often state they heard a 'pop' as the ligament ruptured. It causes pain, swelling and instability. On examination the anterior draw test is positive.

Patella tendon rupture is a less common injury. This would lead to an upward displacement of the patella, and an inability to extend the knee joint and inability to 'straight leg raise'.

Suprapatella effusion is caused by a collection of fluid within the suprapatella bursa. This can occur following injury to the knee. It would cause swelling and if it is large enough may restrict the movement of the joint. On examination there would be a positive patella tap.

30. B
Osteosarcoma

Osteosarcoma is the most common primary malignant bone tumour. It mainly occurs in adolescents, but can also occur secondary to Paget's disease and irradiation of the bone. Osteosarcomas arise from the metaphysis of the long bone and a common site is around the knee. An X-ray of the osteosarcoma would show bone destruction and new bone formation (known as 'sunray spicules'), along with uplifting of the periostium (known as Codman's triangle).

Ewing's sarcoma is a rare primary bone tumour that occurs in children and forms from the round cells of the long bones. Classic radiographic findings include bone destruction along with concentric layers of new bone formation (known as the 'onion ring sign').

Giant cell tumours are also known as osteoclastomas and are rare tumours that are characterised by multinucleate giant cells. They mainly occur in patients between 20–45 years old and form around the epiphysis of the bones. The knee is a common site for them to form. These tumours often progress slowly and X-rays of the area would show osteolysis and may show pathological fractures.

Secondary metastases to the bone are the most common cause of a malignant bone tumour. These classically occur from primary tumours arising from the: breast, lung, thyroid, prostate and kidney. Typically thyroid and renal metastases form lytic lesions, prostate metastases form sclerotic lesions, and breast and lung metastases form mixed lesions. Although this is a classic presentation, in reality it varies a lot.

Osgood-Schlatter disease is a condition that occurs in adolescents. It is due to ossification of the tibial tuberosity apophysitis, which is thought to occur following repeated traction. This leads to inflammation and the tuberosity becomes enlarged and tender. It is associated with physical overactivity. The enlargement of the tibial tuberosity can be seen on radiographs. It causes tenderness and pain that is worsened by contraction of the quadriceps.

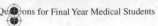

31. D
Menarche at 10 years old

An early menarche is a risk factor for breast cancer. The average age for menarche in the United Kingdom is 12.5 years old. Other risk factors for breast cancer include: late menopause (>50 years old), nulliparity, not breastfeeding, use of the combined oral contraceptive pill, hormone replacement therapy and obesity. The main reason that these are risk factors is that they all lead to increased oestrogen exposure, which is thought to increase the risk of developing breast cancer.

Other risk factors include age, family history, BRCA genes, and exposure to radiation (such as computed tomography [CT] scans and radiotherapy).

Palliative Medicine and Oncology Questions

1. A patient with terminal, widely disseminated metastatic breast cancer is starting to deteriorate. She starts to become restless. She already has a syringe driver set up. Which of the following drugs should be added to treat her agitation?

A. Haloperidol
B. Midazolam
C. Olanzapine
D. Amitriptyline
E. Oxycodone

2. A 70-year-old with prostate cancer and bone metastases is brought into hospital by his carer due to worsening confusion. He had been complaining of a stomach cramps, constipation and nausea. His carer also reported that he was drinking a lot more than normal recently. Examination was unremarkable. Which of the following treatments should be initiated first?

A. 1 litre of 0.9% saline STAT
B. 1 litre of 0.9% saline over 1 hour with intravenous furosemide
C. Intravenous Pamidronate
D. Fluid restriction
E. Tolvaptan

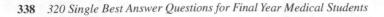
3. A patient currently on an intensive chemotherapy regime is suffering from severe nausea and vomiting. She is already taking ondansetron, cyclizine and metoclopramide. She is also experiencing abdominal pain from liver metastases that are causing the hepatic capsule to be stretched. Which of the following could be added to improve her symptoms?

A. Risperidone
B. Domperidone
C. Dexamethasone
D. Lanzoprazole
E. Cinnarizine

4. An 80-year-old lady currently takes 160 mg of modified release morphine sulfate twice a day and also 40 mg of oramorph four times a day, to control her pain. She is admitted to hospital due to a deterioration of her symptoms. A syringe driver is set up to control her symptoms and also as a precaution in case she can't swallow her oral medications. How much subcutaneous morphine should be written up to control her breakthrough pain?

A. 20 mg
B. 40 mg
C. 80 mg
D. 120 mg
E. 240 mg

5. An elderly man with a past medical history of Lewy body dementia is currently in a care home due to his family being unable to care for him. One night he becomes increasingly confused and begins to shout and get aggressive towards the staff. Which of the following is the most suitable drug to use as a sedative?

A. Haloperidol
B. Lorazepam
C. Zopiclone
D. Trazodone
E. Hydroxyzine

6. A 70-year-old man with an aggressive malignancy is prescribed 60 mg of modified release morphine sulfate twice a day and also given oramorph to treat his breakthrough pain. He has been taking opiates for a while to control his pain. Which of the following drugs should also be prescribed along with his new medications?

A. Movicol
B. Senna
C. Cyclizine
D. Metoclopramide
E. Naloxone

7. A 50-year-old lady presents to her doctor with a feeling of worsening abdominal pain, bloating and early satiety following her meals. She also reports unexplained weight loss that has occurred over the last two months. She has a body mass index (BMI) of 30 and has never been pregnant. Her family history includes her mother and grandmother having breast cancer, which was diagnosed at both 30 and 32 respectively. Her doctor suspects an underlying malignancy. Which of the following tumour markers could be used to monitor her treatment?

A. CA 125
B. CA 19-9
C. CA 15-3
D. Carcinoembryonic antigen (CEA)
E. Human epidermal growth factor receptor 2 (HER-2)

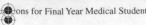

8. A 45-year-old lady is diagnosed with breast cancer. She has a core biopsy, which reveals a poorly differentiated tumour that appears aggressive. On testing it is negative for both oestrogen and progesterone receptors but tests positive for human epidermal growth factor receptor 2 (HER-2). She is started on trastuzumab. Which of the following is she at risk of developing?

A. Peripheral neuropathy
B. Deafness
C. Renal failure
D. Dilated cardiomyopathy
E. Endometrial cancer

9. A 70-year-old man with a terminal diagnosis visits his doctor for a review of his medication. He is currently taking citalopram, paracetamol, naproxen, omeprazole and doxazosin. He is still complaining of pain so his doctor prescribes him tramadol. A few days later he develops a fever, sweating, nausea and vomiting and involuntary muscle twitching. What is the most likely diagnosis?

A. Serotonin syndrome
B. Neuroleptic malignant syndrome
C. Jacksonian march
D. Aseptic meningitis
E. Catatonia

10. A 50-year-old female was recently diagnosed with colorectal cancer. Her mother died at the age of 60 as a result of colorectal cancer and her grandmother was previously diagnosed with uterine and ovarian cancer. Which of the following mutated genes is most likely to have caused this patient's colorectal cancer?

A. APC
B. MSH2
C. STK11
D. VHL
E. RET2

11. A palliative patient with oesophageal cancer is referred to the gastroenterologists for an endoscopy and stenting of the oesophagus. During the procedure the patient experiences severe retrosternal chest pain, and begins to vomit. On examination he is found to have surgical emphysema. Which of the following is most useful in confirming the underlying diagnosis?

A. Electrocardiogram (ECG)
B. Chest X-ray
C. Gastrograffin swallow
D. Continued imaging with the endoscope
E. Echocardiogram

12. A 70-year-old male known to have small cell lung cancer presents to hospital following a fall. On examination he is found to have bilateral nystagmus, ataxia and dysarthria; however there are no signs of weakness or loss of sensation. On examination of the eyes there is no papilloedema. The optic disc can be seen clearly. Which of the following is responsible for his symptoms?

A. Anti-Yo antibodies
B. Hypercalcaemia
C. Hyponatraemia
D. Brain metastases
E. Side effect of vincristine

13. An elderly man is brought into hospital following worsening shortness of breath and two days of haemoptysis. His chest X-ray shows bilateral cannon ball metastases to the lungs. What is the most likely source of the pulmonary metastases?

A. Colorectal cancer
B. Renal cell carcinoma
C. Breast cancer
D. Hepatocellular carcinoma
E. Lymphoma

14. A patient who is diagnosed with Hodgkin's lymphoma receives numerous cycles of chemotherapy and finally recovers fully. Several months later he develops gradual worsening dyspnea. On examination fine end inspiratory crepitations can be heard at both lung bases. An X-ray of his chest shows bilateral reticulonodular shadowing and a normal cardiothoracic ratio of less than 50%. Which of the following medications is responsible for his symptoms?

A. Adriamycin
B. Bleomycin
C. Cisplatin
D. Vincristine
E. Rituximab

15. A 65-year-old non-smoker presents to his doctor following a two-month history of a persistent cough, haemoptysis and weight loss. His doctor requests a chest X-ray, which shows a solitary well defined opacity in the periphery of the right lower lobe. Which of the following is the most likely diagnosis?

A. Adenocarcinoma
B. Small cell carcinoma
C. Squamous cell carcinoma
D. Large cell carcinoma
E. Secondary metastases to the lungs

16. Following a diagnosis of breast cancer a patient is prescribed long-term tamoxifen therapy. Which of the following is she at an increased risk of developing?

A. Osteoporosis
B. Ischaemic heart disease
C. Endometrial cancer
D. Migraines
E. Pulmonary fibrosis

17. Which of the following is most likely to be a paraneoplastic syndrome?

A. Polymyositis
B. Myasthenia gravis
C. Coeliac disease
D. Addison's disease
E. Iron deficiency anaemia

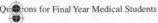

18. A patient with small cell lung cancer is brought into hospital due to confusion. His blood tests show he is hyponatraemic. Which of the following regimes should be used to treat this patient?

A. Fluid restriction
B. 1 litre of 0.9% saline STAT
C. 1 litre of 0.45% saline and 4% dextrose STAT
D. 1 litre of hypotonic saline
E. Desmopressin

19. A patient with suspected neutropenic sepsis is given her second dose of piperacillin/tazobactam. She rapidly develops facial swelling, stridor and wheeze. On examination she is tachycardic, hypotensive and has developed urticaria. Which of the following blood tests can confirm the underlying cause of her symptoms?

A. Neutrophil levels
B. Eosinophil levels
C. Peripheral blood film
D. Serum c-reactive protein (CRP)
E. Serum tryptase levels

20. A palliative patient is currently taking 100 mg of tramadol four times a day, and 65 mg of oramorph four times a day. Her doctor has decided a syringe driver should be set up. How much diamorphine should be added to the syringe driver to control this patient's pain?

A. 60 mg
B. 100 mg
C. 120 mg
D. 240 mg
E. 340 mg

Palliative Medicine and Oncology Answers

1. B
Midazolam

Midazolam is a benzodiazepine, which can be given via a syringe driver in palliative patients to treat agitation. It is the preferred anxiolytic drug in this situation.

Haloperidol is a typical antipsychotic drug that acts as a dopamine D2 receptor antagonist. It can be used in palliative care to treat nausea and vomiting.

Olanzapine is an atypical antipsychotic, and doesn't have a role in palliative care.

Amitriptyline is a tricyclic antidepressant, which can be used to treat neuropathic pain.

Oxycodone is a strong opiate. It has twice the strength of morphine and would be used to treat pain.

2. A
1 litre of 0.9% saline STAT

This patient has developed hypercalcaemia as a result of prostate cancer metastasising to the bone. This presents with polyuria, polydipsia, abdominal pain, anorexia, nausea and vomiting, bone pain, renal stones, depression, psychosis and can also cause hypertension and pancreatitis. Initial treatment is to rehydrate the patient, to protect the kidneys. This is followed by use of intravenous pamidronate, which is a bisphosphonate. The third line treatment is to give furosemide while giving intravenous fluids to increase the renal excretion of calcium, but this can only be started after fluid resuscitation.

Fluid restriction is used to treat patients who are in heart failure or end stage renal failure requiring dialysis and are retaining fluid. It can also be used in patients who develop syndrome of inappropriate antidiuretic hormone (ADH) secretion (SIADH). Tolvaptan is a vaptan drug, which is also used in SIADH, and is a vasopressin/ADH receptor antagonist.

3. C
Dexamethasone

Dexamethasone is a potent corticosteroid. It is very effective in treating patients who are suffering from nausea and vomiting, as a result of chemotherapy treatment. This patient is already taking ondansetron (a serotonin 5-HT3 receptor antagonist), cyclizine (H1 receptor antagonist) and metoclopramide (a D2 receptor antagonist).

Therefore adding domperidone (which is also a D2 receptor antagonist) wouldn't help. Cinnarizine is an antiemetic, which acts as a H1 receptor antagonist. It is mainly used for motion sickness and vertigo.

Risperidone is an atypical antipsychotic, and is not used as an antiemetic and lanzoprazole is a proton pump inhibitor. Neither have a role in treating chemotherapy-induced nausea and vomiting.

This patient is also experiencing pain from liver metastases. This pain is induced by the liver metastases causing the liver capsule to stretch. The most effective treatment for this is to give dexamethasone to reduce the inflammation and oedema around the liver metastases and hence reduce the stretching of the liver capsule.

4. C
80 mg

The dose for breakthrough pain is one sixth of the daily dose of morphine being used to control pain. This patient is currently taking 320 mg of modified release morphine sulfate and 160 mg of oramorph daily. This is a total of 480 mg of morphine per day. One sixth of 480 mg is 80 mg.

5. B
Lorazepam

Lorazepam is a short acting benzodiazepine, which can be used to sedate patients. The other drug listed here that can be used for sedation is haloperidol. However haloperidol is contraindicated in patients with Lewy body dementia or Parkinson's disease. It acts as a dopamine receptor antagonist. These patients are already dopamine depleted, and use of this drug could precipitate a crisis, where patients become extremely rigid and unable to move. Therefore the best option is lorazepam.

Zopiclone belongs to a group known as Z-drugs and is a non-benzodiazepine hypnotic used to treat insomnia. It is not used for sedation on the wards.

Trazodone is a tricyclic antidepressant drug. It can be used in patients who are depressed and also have insomnia. It is given at night and like other tricyclic antidepressants it has a sedating effect and can help aid sleep.

Hydroxyzine is a first generation antihistamine. It crosses the blood brain barrier and therefore can cause drowsiness. It can also be used to aid sleep.

6. B
Senna

The main side effect of opiates is constipation. This is because they bind to and block receptors within the myenteric plexus and reduce the activity of the smooth muscle in the bowel. This is best combated by use of pro-kinetic laxatives, such as senna, which act to increase bowel movements.

Movicol is an osmotic laxative, which acts by pulling water into the intestines. This increases the bulk of the faeces and thus stimulates bowel contractions and movement.

Other side effects of opiates are nausea, vomiting and puritis. Cyclizine and metoclopramide are both antiemetics. One of these may be prescribed on an 'as required basis' when opiates are first used. Opiates can cause nausea and vomiting in patients who are 'opiate-naive', as they haven't used opiates before, so their body isn't used to their effects. Nausea and vomiting are less likely in patients that have used opiates for a long time.

Naloxone is an opiate receptor antagonist, which is used to counteract the effects of an opiate overdose.

7. A
CA 125

This patient has developed ovarian cancer. Ovarian cancer presents very non-specifically. Symptoms include bloating, abdominal distention, early satiety, loss of appetite, weight loss, change in bowel habit/new onset of irritable bowel syndrome in patients over 50 years old and increased urinary frequency.

Risk factors for ovarian cancer include nulliparity, early menarche, late menopause, family history and lack of use of the pill. This lady has two relatives that were diagnosed with breast cancer at a young age. The likelihood of these patients having the BRCA1/2 gene is very high. This gene is associated with both breast and ovarian cancer. Serous cystadenomas are the most common type of ovarian cancer, and their tumour marker is CA 125.

CA 19-9 is found in pancreatic cancer, CA 15-3 is found in breast cancer, CEA is found in colorectal cancer, and HER-2 is found in breast cancer.

8. D
Dilated cardiomyopathy

Use of transtuzumab (Herceptin) is associated with causing a dilated cardiomyopathy. The anthracycline chemotherapeutic agents, such as doxorubicin, can also cause a dilated cardiomyopathy.

Peripheral neuropathy can be caused by vincristine and cisplatin.

Renal failure and deafness can be caused by cisplatin.

Endometrial cancer can occur as a result of tamoxifen use.

9. A
Serotonin syndrome

This is a condition caused by excessive serotonin. It can occur as a result of high doses of antidepressants, co-prescribing different antidepressants, use of recreational drugs such as 3,4-methylenedioxymethamphetamine (MDMA), and also by co-prescribing tramadol with antidepressant (such as citalopram). Serotonin syndrome presents with tachycardia, shivering, sweating, nausea, vomiting, diarrhoea, dilated pupils, myoclonus, hyper-reflexia and can progress to cause seizures.

Neuroleptic malignant syndrome occurs due to co-prescribing different antipsychotic drugs, which results in excessive blockade of the dopamine receptors. It causes hyperthermia, rigidity, extrapyramidal signs (tremor and bradykinesia), and autonomic dysfunction (tachycardia, sweating, urinary incontinence).

Jacksonian march is a type of simple partial/focal seizure whereby the seizure activity begins distally in the limb, and spreads to the rest of that side of the body. It often begins at the fingers as a tingling sensation, followed by uncontrolled movements that then spread up the arm. The patient remains conscious throughout.

Aseptic meningitis is inflamation of the meninges, without the presence of a pyogenic bacterial infection. It presents with classic signs of meningism such as headache, neck stiffness, photophobia, phonophobia, nausea and vomiting. Causes include viral meningitis, autoimmune disease (systemic lupus erythematosus [SLE], sarcoidosis, Bechet's disease), neoplastic disease and drugs non-steroidal anti-inflammatory drugs [NSAIDs], amoxicillin, isoniazid, azathioprine, methotrexate).

Catatonia is a neurogenic motor disorder characterised by a state of stupor. It is associated with schizophrenia, bipolar disorder, post-traumatic stress disorder and depression. It presents with a loss of motor skills, rigidity, repetitive stereotyped movements and waxy flexibility.

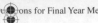

10. B
MSH2

This patient has hereditary non-polyposis colorectal cancer (HNPCC), also known as Lynch disease. This is due to an autosomal dominant mutation in MSH2, MLH1 or PMS2. There are two types of HNPCC. Type 1 causes colorectal cancer and also cancer of the uterus, ovaries, stomach, renal pelvis, and small gut. Type 2 causes colorectal cancer and pancreatic cancer.

APC gene mutations cause familial adenomatous polyposis. This condition is also autosomal dominant and leads to multiple adenomatous polyps forming in the colon, and is one of the greatest risk factors for colorectal cancer. Many patients require a total colectomy as curative treatment.

STK11 causes Peutz–Jeghers syndrome, which is also autosomal dominant, and presents with pigmented macules on the lips and oral mucosa. It is characterised by formation of multiple benign hamartomatous polyps in the gastrointestinal tract. These can lead to bleeding; intussusception and can also become cancerous.

VHL causes von Hippel-Lindau syndrome, which is an autosomal dominant condition, that causes multiple tumours to develop. It can cause bilateral renal cell carcinomas, retinal and cerebellar haemangioblastomas (hence it can cause visual impairment and cerebellar signs) and also phaeochromocytoma.

RET2 causes multiple endocrine neoplasia type 2 (MEN2). This can be either MEN2a, which presents with medullary thyroid carcinoma, phaeochromocytoma and parathyroid hyperplasia; or MEN2b which causes medullary thyroid carcinoma, phaeochromocytoma, marfanoid appearance and mucosal neuromas.

11. C
Gastrograffin swallow

This patient has oesophageal rupture. This can be iatrogenic such as in endoscopy, as a result of penetrating trauma, ingestion of corrosive agents, invasive malignancy, or violent vomiting (also known as Boerhaave syndrome). It presents with shock, fever, odynophagia, vomiting, chest pain and surgical emphysema. Gastrograffin swallow can be utilized to make the diagnosis. Barium swallow is more accurate, but is too irritant to the mediastinum and therefore not used. Gastrograffin is a water-soluble contrast and less irritant.

ECG would be first line if this patient were having a myocardial infarction. This is less likely due to the presence of surgical emphysema.

Chest X-ray would reveal any chest pathology. In oesophageal rupture it may show a widened mediastinum and pleural effusion, but these findings are not specific to oesophageal rupture.

Endoscopy is now contraindicated in this patient as it can extend the perforation and introduce more air into the mediastinum.

Echocardiogram would provide detailed imaging of the heart. It is not currently indicated in this patient.

12. A
Anti-Yo antibodies

This patient has developed paraneoplastic cerebellar degeneration as a result of his small cell carcinoma. Anti-Yo antibodies are responsible for this. This would present with bilateral cerebellar signs.

Brain metastases can occur in lung cancer but are likely to also cause weakness and changes in sensation, as they wouldn't just be confined to the cerebellum. They would also lead to a raised intracranial pressure thus causing papilloedema. Brain metastases are possible, but to occur bilaterally to the cerebellum, and not affect the cortex at all is very unlikely.

Hypercalcaemia can occur as a result of bone metastases. This would present with bone pain, pathological fractures, renal calculi, polyuria, polydipsia, abdominal pain, anorexia and depression.

Hyponatraemia can be caused by syndrome of inappropriate antidiuretic hormone (ADH) secretion (SIADH) as a result of small cell lung cancer. This would present with confusion, weakness, headaches and seizures.

Vincristine is a chemotherapeutic drug used in treatment of small cell lung cancers, but its main side effect is peripheral neuropathy.

13. B
Renal cell carcinoma

The three cancers that commonly metastasise to the lungs are breast cancer, renal cell carcinoma and colorectal cancer. The two causes of cannon ball metastases are renal cell carcinomas and much less commonly testicular teratomas.

Renal cell carcinomas are likely to present with haematuria, loin pain and weight loss. Investigations may show a raised blood pressure and polycythaemia.

14. B
Bleomycin

Bleomycin is a chemotherapeutic drug that acts by causing breaks in DNA strands. Its main side effect is pulmonary fibrosis, which is what this patient has developed. It presents with a dry cough, worsening breathlessness and on examination there is reduced chest expansion and bilateral basal fine end inspiratory crepitations.

Adriamycin is also known as doxorubicin and acts by preventing the action of topoisomerase II and the synthesis of DNA. It can cause a dilated cardiomyopathy.

Cisplatin acts by the platinum component binding to bases, thus affecting DNA synthesis. Its side effects include nephrotoxicity, neurotoxicity, ototoxicity, nausea and vomiting.

Vincristine is a vinca alkaloid and binds to tubulin dimers thus inhibiting mitosis. Its main side effect is a peripheral neuropathy. It can also cause hyponatraemia and constipation.

Rituximab is a monoclonal antibody against the CD20 component of B-cells. It is used in both treatment of lymphoma and auto-immune diseases. Its use causes immunosuppression, which can lead to infection.

15. A
Adenocarcinoma

This patient has an underlying diagnosis of lung cancer. The most common cause of lung cancer in non-smokers is an adenocarcinoma. These are classically found in the peripheries of the lungs.

Squamous cell carcinomas are the most common cause of lung cancer in smokers. These present with large central masses, which can cavitate.

Small cell carcinomas often present before they can be seen on a chest X-ray. They are aggressive cancers that metastasise early and are associated with a number of paraneoplastic syndromes.

Large cell carcinomas are a group of undifferentiated carcinomas. These form between 5–10% of all lung cancers.

Secondary metastases to the lungs would more commonly present with multiple lesions in the lungs and also with signs and symptoms from the primary tumour. Causes include breast, renal and colon cancer.

16. C
Endometrial cancer

Tamoxifen is a selective oestrogen receptor modulator, which activates the oestrogen receptors in the bone, but not in the breast tissue. It is prescribed as secondary prophylaxis in patients who have been treated for breast cancer, and who have not been through the menopause. Its side effects include venous thromboembolism, facial flushing, deranged liver function tests, vaginal bleeding and increased risk of endometrial cancer. The reason it causes an increased risk of endometrial cancer is that there is unopposed oestrogen activity, which causes hyperplasia of the endometrial lining.

Osteoporosis is a side effect of aromatase inhibitors such as letrozole. Aromatase inhibitors are used as secondary prophylaxis for breast cancer in patients who have been through the menopause. In postmenopausal women, oestrogen is produced in adipose tissue, by the conversion of androgens to oestrogen, through the activity of aromatase enzymes. This is inhibited by letrozole.

Ischaemic heart disease is a side effect of fluorouracil (5-FU), which is a chemotherapy drug used to treat breast cancer.

Migraines are a common side effect of hormonal contraceptives.

Pulmonary fibrosis can be caused by bleomycin, which is another chemotherapeutic drug.

17. A
Polymyositis

A paraneoplastic syndrome is a set of signs or symptoms that occur as a result of a particular malignancy, but not due to the mass effect of the tumour, or due to the effect of metastases. They are often mediated by hormones secreted by the tumour, or the immune system response to the presence of a tumour.

Polymyositis is an autoimmune connective tissue disease, which causes inflammation of the muscles. It typically presents with progressive painful muscle weakness. Other signs and symptoms may include arthralgia, fever, Raynaud's phenomenon, and interstitial lung fibrosis and myocardial involvement causing a myocarditis. It is a paraneoplastic syndrome. Cancers that are known to cause it include small cell lung cancer, bladder cancer and non-Hodgkin's lymphoma.

Myasthenia gravis is an autoimmune condition caused by anti-acetylcholine receptor antibodies, which are present at the neuromuscular junction. This is not a paraneoplastic syndrome, but Lambert-Eaton syndrome can occur as a paraneoplastic syndrome. This is a similar condition caused by anti-voltage gated calcium channel antibodies.

Coeliac disease is not a paraneoplastic syndrome, but is associated with a higher risk of developing certain cancers in the future. These include gastrointestinal T-cell lymphoma, gastric, oesophageal, bladder, breast and brain cancers.

Addison's disease is also known as primary adrenal insufficiency. This doesn't classically occur as a paraneoplastic syndrome, but can be caused by metastases to the adrenal glands. Cancers that do so include lung, breast and renal cancers.

18. A
Fluid restriction

This patient has developed syndrome of inappropriate antidiuretic hormone (ADH) secretion (SIADH), which has led to him developing hyponatraemia. This is a paraneoplastic syndrome caused by the neuroendocrine cells that make up the small cell lung cancer. Treatment is fluid restriction and use of drugs called vaptans. These act as ADH receptor antagonists. Giving fluids in this condition would only cause it to worsen.

Desmopressin is an ADH analogue and would also worsen the condition. Desmopressin is used to treat cranial diabetes insipidus, which is caused by a lack of ADH.

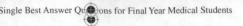

19. E
Serum tryptase levels

This patient has developed anaphylaxis due to a penicillin allergy. Tryptase is an enzyme released by mast cells, and an increase in its level is highly suggestive that the underlying diagnosis is due to an immunologically mediated reaction.

Eosinophils are also likely to be raised in patients who have allergies, but the recommended test is to use tryptase levels, as these would rise a lot faster. Eosinophils can also be raised in asthma, parasitic infections, and skin conditions (eczema, psoriasis, bullous pemphigus and erythema multiforme).

Neutrophils can be raised in bacterial infections, chronic myeloid leukaemia, inflammation (myocardial infarction, vasculitis, inflammatory bowel disease), corticosteroid use, disseminated malignancy and burns.

CRP is an acute phase protein, which is raised in almost any cause of inflammation. It is commonly raised in infections, inflammatory bowel disease, and rheumatoid arthritis.

Peripheral blood films are used to help diagnose a variety of haematological conditions. They are used if a haematological malignancy is suspected.

20. B
100 mg

Tramadol can be converted to oral morphine by dividing the dosage by 10. Therefore the daily dosage of oral morphine this patient is having is: $(100 \text{ mg} \times 4)/10 + 65 \text{ mg} \times 4 = 300 \text{ mg}$.

This patient is having a total of 300 mg of oral morphine a day. Oral morphine can be converted to subcutaneous diamorphine by dividing the dose by 3. Therefore she requires 100 mg of diamorphine in her syringe driver.

Printed in the United States
By Bookmasters